The Bedford Murder
An Evidence-Based Clinical Mystery

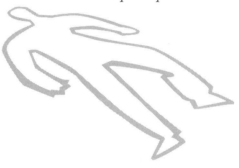

The Bedford Murder

An Evidence-Based Clinical Mystery

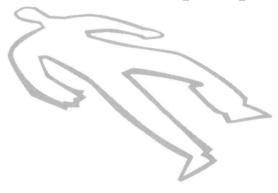

Marshall Godwin MD, CCFP, FCFP
Associate Professor and Director of Research
Department of Family Medicine
Director, Centre for Studies in Primary Care
Queen's University, Kingston, Ontario, Canada

Geoffrey Hodgetts MD, CCFP, FCFP
Associate Professor, Queen's University
Kingston, Ontario, Canada

HANLEY & BELFUS, INC.
An Imprint of Elsevier

HANLEY & BELFUS, INC.
An Imprint of Elsevier

The Curtis Center
Independence Square West
Philadelphia, Pennsylvania 19106

Note to the reader: Although the information in this book has been carefully reviewed for correctness of dosage and indications, neither the authors nor the editors nor the publisher can accept any legal responsibility for any errors or omissions that may be made. Neither the publisher nor the editors make any warranty, expressed or implied, with respect to the material contained herein. Before prescribing any drug, the reader must review the manufacturer's current product information (package inserts) for accepted indications, absolute dosage recommendations, and other information pertinent to the safe and effective use of the product described.

Library of Congress Control Number: 2003101348

THE BEDFORD MURDER
AN EVIDENCE-BASED CLINICAL MYSTERY   ISBN 1-56053-565-2

Last digit is the print number: 9 8 7 6 5 4 3 2 1

Family Tree

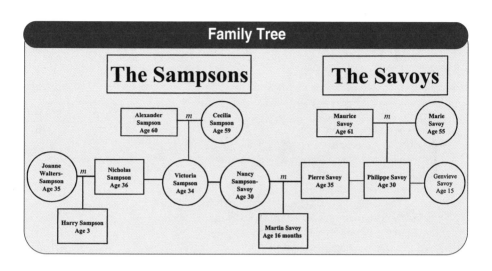

The Sampsons

Alexander Sampson Age 60 — m — Cecilia Sampson Age 59

Joanne Walters-Sampson Age 35 — m — Nicholas Sampson Age 36

Victoria Sampson Age 34

Nancy Sampson-Savoy Age 30

Harry Sampson Age 3

The Savoys

Maurice Savoy Age 61 — m — Marie Savoy Age 55

Pierre Savoy Age 35

Philippe Savoy Age 30

Genvieve Savoy Age 15

Nancy Sampson-Savoy Age 30 — m — Pierre Savoy Age 35

Martin Savoy Age 16 months

Other Significant Characters in the Story

Dr. Leslie Sharpe	the clinical sleuth in the story
Amy Stephens	the victim whose body was found in the trunk of a car
Beatrice Stephens	Amy Stephens' mother
Joan Walters	Joanne Walters-Sampson's aunt; Matthew Walters' sister
Matthew Walters	Joanne Walters' father
Sean FitzPatrick	a police officer in Bedford
Robert Stensen	driver and butler for the Sampson family
Stefan Richard	driver and butler for the Savoy family
Joey Hynes and Leo Nash	a couple of ex-cons and crime underworld sorts
Jenny Ling	a nurse at the Bedford Family Medicine Clinic
Dr. Jonathon Simple	Dr. Sharpe's colleague and friend
Dr. Gerald Wells and his wife Margaret	another physician at the clinic

ACT III

ACT IV

PREFACE

First and foremost this book is about evidence. It is a murder mystery and the evidence must be considered to determine who-done-it; it also models the process of Evidence-Based Medicine (EBM) in clinical practice; and finally it is a book of evidence-based clinical pearls. It is about critical appraisal, clinical practice, and entertainment all rolled into one. And it works!

For those not familiar with the process of incorporating EBM into practice, the book models the five steps of EBM: i) asking a clinical question, ii) finding sources of information to answer the question, iii) critically appraising that information, iv) making a practice decision based on the critically appraised evidence, v) and then reflecting, after a period of time, on the effect of that practice decision.

The book is based on clinical cases presenting to a family doctor's office. It deals with diabetes, hypertension, depression, oral contraception, tennis elbow, urinary tract infections, gastroesophageal reflux and much more. The clinical pearls are evidence-based, succinct, and pertinent.

And spun through the book is a story, a murder mystery. The main character is a young family doctor who is intent on finding out why one of her patients has suddenly disappeared. The disappearance is affecting many of the patients in her practice, especially the missing man's family members. A fishing trip, a love affair from the past, and two families of some means who are linked by marriage but with little else in common, all play a part. As the clues mount, the family doctor, as well as the reader, try to determine from the evidence just what is going on.

Each clinical encounter in this book is followed by a number of clinical questions that arise from it. We (the authors) have done a detailed literature search to identify the best evidence to answer these questions, but the reader needs to consider what other information or evidence he or she is aware of, and from which sources, that might also be used to help answer the questions. We have critically appraised the articles we are citing and have come to conclusions based on the evidence, as we see it. Readers need to decide if they agree. Perhaps the conclusions we arrive at are inappropriate for the context of the reader's clinical practice. We have made decisions about how the family doctor in the book applied the evidence to her clinical situation. Readers should decide whether they agree with this and whether they would apply the results in the same way or a different way.

It is useful to recognize that there are five types of clinical questions asked in this book. They are questions of diagnosis, therapy, harm, prognosis, and etiology.

Diagnosis questions are about factors or tests that help with diagnosis. These tests may be laboratory or imaging investigations, but they may also be features on history and physical examination. Generally, sensitivity and specificity are addressed. They may be studies that look at the accuracy of a rapid screening test for diagnosing a specific condition. Generally, the test is compared to a gold standard (e.g., when determining how well the urine dipstick test detects urinary tract infection, its accuracy would be compared to the gold standard of a urine culture; or a diagnosis may ask how accurately the presence of green sputum on history predicts the presence of pneumonia on chest x-ray).

Therapy questions are about the effectiveness of therapy. They may be about a drug or a nonpharmacological therapy. Generally these questions ask about the value of a treatment at decreasing symptoms, curing a disease, preventing further morbidity, or decreasing mortality.

Harm questions are about the potential for harmful effects of drugs or other treatments or the potential for harmful effects of diagnostics tests. They may also relate to the potentially harmful effects of environmental substances on disease, but here the boundary between etiology and harm begins to blur. In this book the questions of harm generally refer to harmful effects of treatments or diagnostic tests.

Prognosis questions relate to the ability to predict the outcome of a given disease or condition based on certain features of the disease or of the individual. Perhaps men who smoke and are hypertensive may be more likely to die within 5 years of contracting a certain condition than are women who do not smoke and are not hypertensive.

Etiology questions are about factors that are causally related to the development of a specific condition or disease. Does stress cause this condition? Which bacteria are most likely to cause infection in this location? This type of question can be similar to a question about harm.

There are a number of types of research studies that may be conducted to answer the different types of questions. Depending on the methodology used, these studies can be ranked based on the strength of their design and their ability to accurately answer the type of question. This has led to a concept of Levels of Evidence whereby (for questions of therapy, harm, and etiology) well done randomized controlled trials are considered to produce very high levels of evidence and case-series studies to produce a significantly lower level of evidence. Expert opinion that is not based on good research is the lowest level of evidence of all. Detailed information on Levels of Evidence can be found at http://www.eboncall.co.uk/content/levels.html

We used a "real-life" approach in the book; that is, we asked the clinical question and then went in search of the evidence rather than finding a good article and concocting a clinical scenario around it. There are many sources and types of information or "evidence"—randomized controlled trials, cohort studies, case-control studies, studies evaluating the sensitivity and specificity of a test, or descriptive studies, to name a few. These are different types of studies providing evidence of varying quality. Many times the best available evidence was of low quality. So we used whatever evidence and information we could find to provide the best care to the patient.

For members of the College of Family Physicians of Canada

This book has been endorsed by the College of Family Physicians of Canada (CFPC) as being appropriate for family practice in Canada. Information and forms are provided in the appendix about how you can obtain up to 10 MAINPRO-C credits as you work though the clinical cases.

We trust that you will see our book as an educational resource. We hope you will find it useful, not only for its clinical content, but because it helped you better understand concepts of EBM and critical appraisal. And most of all, we hope you enjoy the story.

Marshall Godwin MD CCFP

Geoffrey Hodgetts MD CCFP

Bedford has a population of 40,000 souls, more or less. Most are reasonably happy; others spend their lives in what seems like eternal misery. Envy, vengeance, hatred, and arrogance live side by side with love, patience, and humility. Bedford is big enough to be called a city, yet hardly metropolitan; it is small enough to feel a kinship with the surrounding farming communities, yet is not quite rural itself. Its terrain is flat, and its streets are laid out in a perfect criss-cross pattern. Flying overhead and looking down you can imagine playing tic-tac-toe. It is a hundred kilometers to the nearest mountain to ski, and to the nearest river with rapids to shoot. It is just as far to the nearest real city where one could experience a real nightlife. The middle of nowhere you might think! Yet in many ways it is typical of a small city in the lowlands of the Great Lakes basin in southern Ontario.

Who would live in Bedford? Certainly not those who want a fast city life; yet also not those who like the smell of the farm or the sound of rapids in the northern wilderness. As the country people surrounding Bedford come into town for short and necessary shopping excursions, so Bedfordians leave. Leave for the larger city for the weekend, or for a canoe trip up north. Like the fishing trip to Labrador that ended somewhat mysteriously last week. But more of that later!

Who would live in Bedford? You do! You arrived five years ago, landing at its small airport shortly after that game of tic-tac-toe. Single, smart, and fresh out of a family medicine residency, you were ready to take on the world. You are still single, though maybe not for long; still smart, though not as smart as you thought you were; and there is still lots of illness out there to keep you busy.

All families are important in Bedford, but two families in particular seem to dominate the others: the Sampsons and the Savoys. It seems everyone in Bedford is related to these two families in some way; or at least has had their lives affected by them. One is of English origin, the other French; a microcosm of Canada. Both are families of some means; both commanding and sometimes deserving respect; both with closets so full of skeletons they are bursting at the seams!

The Sampsons have been lawyers and politicians in Bedford for generations. Theirs is old money. Alexander Sampson owns the largest law firm in town and has served two terms as mayor over the years. Cecilia, his wife, trained as a nurse but does mainly charity work now. They are in their late fifties, they have raised three children, two daughters and a son, and have four grandchildren. Alex has four sisters living in town, married with children and grandchildren. Cecilia comes from a large family of 8 siblings. All but two live in Bedford or surrounds. Nieces, nephews, aunts and uncles abound. Directly or through marriage many people in Bedford are related to the Sampsons. You have to be careful what you say and to whom you say it.

The Savoys moved here just 30 years ago. They are business people and have prospered. They own the local car dealership, the largest supermarket, and recently got into contract construction work. Maurice Savoy and his wife Marie have two sons and a daughter, and all are involved in the family businesses. Like the Sampsons they have extended family, being from large families themselves, but most of their family live in other cities or provinces. Their son Pierre is married to Nancy Sampson, Alex and Cecilia Sampson's daughter. They live in Bedford.

By now you know many of the interrelationships of the people in this town. You have been there during times of grief, during marriage breakups, and illness. They have confided in you, angered you, thanked you, and blamed you. You are Dr. Leslie Sharpe, and you are about to start your clinic for the day.

ACT I

Cecilia's Distress
(Diabetes Mellitus)

Cecilia has been your patient for 5 years. She was diagnosed with high blood pressure 10 years ago, 5 years before your arrival in Bedford. Two years ago, you diagnosed diabetes mellitus after she had two episodes of monilial vaginitis and was feeling tired. You did the usual things. You talked to her about exercise and diet and the fact that starches and sugars needed to be considered. You sent her to the dietitian at the hospital for further dietary training, and you ordered all the appropriate laboratory tests to look for end-organ damage and other risk factors for cardiovascular disease.

She tried diet management at first and lost 5 lb in the first month, but by 3 months she had gained it back. Her blood glucose values were 12–14 mmol/L, so you started her on glyburide, 2.5 mg daily, which was increased over time to 5 mg twice daily. Recently her fasting blood glucose values have been 7.8–8.4 mmol/L.

Cecilia had gone to the laboratory this morning to have a fasting blood glucose done. When you tell her the result was 11.8 mmol/L, she cries and wonders if it could be due to stress. You listen as Cecilia tells her story.

Nicholas, her son who is known as Nick generally, had been on a fishing trip in Labrador with Pierre Savoy. Pierre Savoy is Cecilia's son-in-law; he married Cecilia's daughter Nancy 5 years earlier. The men left for their 2-week trip just 2 weeks ago. They drove in separate cars to Toronto, left their cars in the parking garage at the airport, and flew to Goose Bay, Labrador. Cecilia knew they arrived safely because Nick called Joanne, his wife, after they arrived in Goose Bay. He called again yesterday from Goose Bay before getting on the plane to fly home. Joanne had said he was excited about the wonderful trip they had.

Pierre arrived home last evening, but Nick hasn't arrived yet and hasn't called. Pierre said the last time he saw him was in the distance when Nick was opening the trunk of his car to put his gear in. They had parked several rows apart in the garage. Pierre had left ahead of Nick, and during the 2-hour trip home to Bedford he hadn't noticed Nick's car behind him at any point. Alexander Sampson, Nick's father, had called the police, but there were no reports of unidentified accident victims. Alex was on his way to Toronto to see if the car was still in the parking garage. Pierre was with him. The whole family is so worried.

Cecilia had decided to keep her appointment because she needed to talk to you. She always felt better after discussing problems with you because you are such a good listener and you don't rush her. She also wondered if a tranquilizer might help her because she is so upset and is unable to sleep.

You tell her you understand how awful she must feel and that her blood glucose value might be due to the increased stress. You suggest she not use tranquilizers at this point but wait and see what Alex and Pierre are able to find out. You suggest she go home and rest and come back in to see you anytime she needs to. You also tell her you want to see her in 1 week to recheck her blood glucose. She thanks you for your kindness and goes home.

Before you see your next patient, you reflect on the strange story you just heard. It had not hit the news yet, but you suspect it will be in the evening paper. Why would Nick just disappear like that? According to Cecilia, he seemed upbeat when he called his wife before leaving Goose Bay to come home. Given the fact that he called home twice from Goose Bay, it seemed unlike him not to get in touch with his family—unless he wasn't able to or had good reason not to. You had seen him once or twice in clinic for simple things and when his wife was in labor with their child, 3 years ago. Men in their 30s don't visit physicians much. Oh well, you thought, on with the morning!

Some questions arising from this clinical encounter

1   In a 59-year-old woman with non–insulin-dependent diabetes mellitus on oral hypoglycemic agents and blood glucose values around 8 mmol/L, would intensifying her treatment to decrease the fasting blood glucose further decrease the likelihood of diabetes-related complications and disease?

2   In a 59-year-old woman in acute distress and with insomnia because of a family crisis, would a benzodiazepine be helpful, and what is the risk of dependency?

3   In a 59-year-old woman with non–insulin-dependent diabetes mellitus, would the stress of an acute emotional crisis be likely to result in an elevation of her blood glucose?

Reflection Exercise:

What are your thoughts regarding these questions? Consider them in the context of your own practice. Consider what you might do before you read the evidence.

Citation: UK Prospective Diabetes Study Group. Intensive blood-glucose control with sulphonylureas or insulin compared with conventional treatment and risk of complications in patients with type 2 diabetes. Lancet 1998; 352:837–853.[105]

Study design: Randomized controlled trial, blinded, multicentered, with intention-to-treat analysis.

Sample size: 3867

Study population: Patients throughout the United Kingdom with newly diagnosed diabetes between 1977 and 1991. Age range, 25–65 years; mean age, 53.4 years at time of enrollment; 61% men.

Intervention group (N = 2729; 2729 analyzed): Diet plus glibenclamide (glyburide), chlorpropamide, insulin, or combinations to achieve a goal of fasting blood glucose (FBG) of ≤6 mmol/L. The median FBG achieved in the intervention group was about 7.7 mmol/L, and the median hemoglobin A_{1c} was 7.0%.

Control group (N = 1138; 1138 analyzed): Diet alone to try to keep the FBG <15 mmol/L and the patient free of hyperglycemic symptoms. Medication added to diet if needed to achieve these goals. The median FBG attained in the control group was 9.4 mmol/L over the 11-year follow-up. The median hemoglobin A_{1c} for the 11 years was 7.9%.

Other study details: No significant difference between groups at baseline on weight, blood pressure, smoking, cholesterol levels, or any other of the many assessed parameters. Patients followed for mean of 11.1 years.

The Evidence

Outcome	EER (Intervention)	CER (Conventional)	Relative Risk	ARR	NNTb
Any diabetes-related end point	963 of 2729 (35.3%)	438 of 1138 (38.5%)	0.91 (0.81–1.0)	NA	NA
Diabetes-related deaths	285 of 2729 (10.4%)	129 of 1138 (11.3%)	0.92 (0.75–1.12)	NA	NA
All-cause mortality	489 of 2729 (17.8%)	213 of 1138 (18.7%)	0.95 (0.72–1.10)	NA	NA
Myocardial infarction	387 of 2729 (14.2%)	186 of 1138 (16.3%)	0.87 (0.74–1.03)	NA	NA
Stroke	148 of 2729 (5.4%)	55 of 1138 (4.8%)	0.88 (0.84–1.49)	NA	NA
Amputation or death from PVD	29 of 2729 (1%)	18 of 1138 (1.6%)	0.62 (0.33–1.20)	NA	NA
Microvascular	225 of 2729 (8.2%)	121 of 1138 (10.6%)	0.77 (0.62–0.97)	2.4%	42

EER, experimental event rate; CER, control event rate; ARR, absolute risk reduction; NNTb, number needed to treat to benefit 1 person; NA, not applicable as there is no significant difference; PVD, peripheral vascular disease.

Interpretation: In this study, microvascular complications included retinopathy requiring photocoagulation, vitreous hemorrhage, and fatal or nonfatal renal failure. This was the only outcome that was significantly improved by the intensive treatment. A total of 42 type 2 diabetics would have to receive this intensive treatment for 11 years to prevent 1 from getting a microvascular complication. The absolute risk reduction of a microvascular complication was 2.4% over 11 years. The intensive treatments, whether they involved the use of insulin or oral hypoglycemic agents, did not decrease significantly the likelihood of myocardial infarction, stroke, or peripheral vascular disease. These results are consistent with earlier studies, which showed a benefit only in microvascular conditions, such as retinopathy, neuropathy, and nephropathy.[29,55]

Major hypoglycemic episodes were significantly more common among the intensive treatment group; 1.0% with chlorpropamide, 1.4% with glibenclamide (glyburide), 2.3% with insulin, and 0.7% with diet. One patient in the conventional treatment group died of diabetic coma, one patient in the intensive group (on insulin) died of hypoglycemia. Patients on intensive treatment gained significantly more weight than patients on conventional treatment. This outcome was noted previously.[55]

The FBG and the hemoglobin A_{1c} levels achieved by the intensive treatment group are above the recommended levels in current recommendations, which suggest keeping hemoglobin A_{1c} <7.0%.[2] Most studies comparing intensive with less intensive treatments rarely are able to achieve levels of hemoglobin A_{1c} <7.0%. This may be an unrealistic recommendation given the difficulty in achieving it even in controlled study situations and because the likelihood of further benefit compared with potential harm (hypoglycemia) is low.

Bottom line: Striving to keep a FBG at 7–8 mmol/L and the hemoglobin A_{1c} as close to 7% as possible could be of some benefit to Mrs. Sampson. It would decrease the likelihood of her developing microvascular complications, with a slight but probably acceptable increase in risk of major hypoglycemic episodes.

What did Dr. Sharpe do?

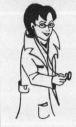

Dr. Sharpe decided to order a hemoglobin A_{1c} test, and if it was >7% or if the FBG continued to be >8 mmol/L on more than an infrequent basis, better control would have to be tried, either by increasing the glyburide or by adding metformin. Which option is best? That's another question!

Reflection Exercise: How does this evidence apply to your practice? Would you apply this evidence to the management of appropriate patients in your practice? How will your practice change?

Preamble

We were struck by the absence of research on the simple questions: "What is the risk of dependency if a patient is started on a benzodiazepine?" and "Does a benzodiazepine help in short-term situational anxiety situations?" The answers to these direct questions are not available as far as we can determine. We found high-level evidence articles on characteristics of long-term benzodiazepine users in general practice,[96] health of long-term benzodiazepine users,[87] risk of car crashes in people taking benzodiazepines,[41] risk of falls in people taking benzodiazepines,[60] benzodiazepine use in the treatment of insomnia,[44] and nonpharmacologic interventions in insomnia.[70] Numerous opinion pieces, descriptive articles, and pharmacology-based articles are available. From all of these, we have pieced together an answer to this question.

Citation: Holbrook AM, Crowther R, Lotter A, et al. Meta-analysis of benzodiazepine use in the treatment of insomnia. Can Med Assoc J 2000; 162:225–233.[44]

Study type: Systematic review with meta-analysis.

Data sources: Cochrane Library, Medline, hand searching of references in articles.

Number of studies: 45

Number of patients: 2672

Time frame: 1979–1993

Article selection criteria: Randomized controlled trials comparing benzodiazepines with placebo or with an alternate drug for effects on insomnia.

Data extraction: Data were collected on study design, conditions treated, patient characteristics, setting and duration of the trial, and outcomes measured.

Article appraisal process: There were multiple independent reviews of the individual articles. Interrater reliability was 98%. Disagreement was resolved by consensus.

Statistical heterogeneity tests? Yes. Heterogeneity tests were nonsignificant for the high-quality studies. It was reasonable to pool the data.

Publication bias testing? Not mentioned.

Other study details: There were 2672 patients in the 45 randomized controlled trials used for analysis. Women comprised 47% of the study patients. Mean age range was 29–82 years. The duration of the studies ranged from 1 day to 6 weeks with a mean duration of 12.2 days. Studies involved flurazepam, temazepam, midazolam, nitrazepam, estazolam, lorazepam, diazepam, brotizolam, quazepam, loprazolam, and flunitrazepam.

The Evidence

Outcome	Mean Difference (Treatment − Placebo) (95% Confidence Interval)	P Value
Sleep latency (time it took to get to sleep) (min)	−4.2 (−0.7–9.2)	NS
Total sleep duration (min)	61.8 (37.4–86.2)	<0.05

Outcome	EER (Benzodiazepine)	CER (Control)	Odds Ratio (95% Confidence Interval)	ARI	NNTh
Side effects	298 of 506 (59%)	222 of 502 (44%)	1.8 (1.4–2.4)	15%	7

NS, not significant; EER, experimental event rate; CER, control event rate; ARI, absolute risk increase, NNTh, number needed to treat to harm 1 person.

Citation: Hemmelgarn B, Suissa S, Huang A, et al. Benzodiazepine use and the risk of motor vehicle crash in the elderly. JAMA 1997; 278:27–31.[41]

Interpretation: This systematic review concludes that compared with placebo, benzodiazepines help people with insomnia sleep longer by approximately 1 hour. They do not help people get to sleep any more quickly. There also are more adverse events reported on benzodiazepines, including drowsiness, dizziness, light-headedness, and cognitive impairment. These events did not lead to a higher discontinuation rate among people taking benzodiazepines. The studies did not look at quality of sleep or quality of life in benzodiazepine users compared with controls. The authors suggest this as an area for research.

Bottom line: Benzodiazepines help insomniacs sleep about 1 hour longer but do not help them get to sleep any faster. Side effects occur but seem to be minor.

Study design: Nested case-control.

Sample size: Difficult to ascertain. There were 5579 cases and 10 controls for each case selected from a subcohort of 13,256 people. An individual in the subcohort could serve as a control more than once, but it had to be on a different day.

Study population: All eligible drivers age 67–84 years in the province of Quebec, Canada, were determined using the computerized driver's license file of the *Societe de l'assurance automobile du Quebec.* This agency is responsible for driver's license registration and recording reports of motor vehicle crashes.

Cases: Cases (5579) were people age 67–84 who had an injurious motor vehicle crash.

Controls: There were 55,790 control person-days (people who did not have a crash on that day).

Exposures of interest: Use of benzodiazepine drugs as determined by computerized pharmacy records. Exposures to short-half-life drug (≤24 hours) and long-half-life drug (>24 hours) were considered separately.

Outcome: Involvement, as a driver, in a motor vehicle crash in which at least one person (not necessarily the driver) sustained bodily injury.

Other study details: Cases were similar to controls with regard to age, residence, and chronic disease score, but cases were more likely to be male, to have been exposed to other central nervous system drugs before their crash, and to have had a previous injurious motor vehicle accident. The raw data had identified 6064 cases (motor crashes) from 224,734 subjects. This baseline cohort rate of 2.6% for motor crashes is what we used to calculate number needed to treat to harm 1 person (NNTh) (from the odds ratios) for benzodiazepine use and the absolute risk increase was then calculated from the NNTh.

The Evidence

Exposure	Cases Involved in Injurious Motor Vehicle Crash	Controls Not Involved in Injurious Motor Vehicle Crash	Adjusted Odds Ratio	ARI	NNTh
On long-half-life benzodiazepines	387 of 3817 (10.1%)	2911 of 38,511 (7.5%)	1.28 (1.12–1.45)	0.7%	132
On short-half-life benzodiazepines	811 of 4241 (19.1%)	8202 of 43,802 (18.7%)	0.96 0.88–1.05	NA	NA

ARI, absolute risk increase; NNTh, number needed to treat to harm 1 person; NA, not applicable as there is no significant difference.

Interpretation: The cases were at higher risk for motor vehicle accidents because they were more likely to be male, to have taken other drugs that affect the central nervous system, and to have had a previous car accident. To control for this, the authors present an adjusted odds ratio, presumable from a logistic regression analysis. The increased risk for injurious accidents remained, after adjustment, for long-half-life benzodiazepines but did not remain significant for short-half-life benzodiazepines.

Bottom line: Benzodiazepines with a long half-life (>24 hours) are more likely to be associated with injurious motor vehicle crashes than placebo in the elderly. You would need to place 132 elderly people on long-half-life benzodiazepine for 1 additional person to have a serious accident.

Overall Conclusion

Benzodiazepines are effective in insomnia[44,69] and are the mainstay for the short-term treatment of anxiety.[1] Short-acting benzodiazepines are probably preferable to the long-acting type because they are less likely to increase the risk of motor vehicle accidents. Short-term and long-term benzodiazepines can increase the risk of falls in people >60 years old (odds ratio, 1.47; 95% confidence interval, 1.23–1.77).[60] Abuse is more likely if benzodiazepines are prescribed to patients with a history of drug abuse.[69] Long-term use (>4 months) results in a significantly increased likelihood of dependence and withdrawal symptoms.[77] The best advice is to use benzodiazepines when it is believed pharmacologic treatment is required for insomnia or anxiety but for short periods (≤4 weeks); use low-dose, short-acting benzodiazepines (e.g., lorazepam, oxazepam); and use with caution in the elderly (>60 years old). Elderly people should be warned of the risk of falls and motor vehicle accidents.

What did Dr. Sharpe do?

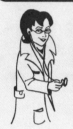

Dr. Sharpe isn't totally against prescribing benzodiazepines and has used short-acting preparations occasionally in the past. Mrs. Sampson is approaching 60 years of age, however, and she has handled stress well in the past. Dr. Sharpe decided to wait and see how she would manage without medications. They chatted for a while, discussing strategies to help relieve stress and anxiety. Do these relaxation and other strategies really work for stress and insomnia? Another question for another day!

Reflection Exercise: How does this evidence apply to your practice? Would you apply this evidence to the management of appropriate patients in your practice? How will your practice change?

Answer to Question 3

Citation: Goetsch VL, Abel JL, Pope MK. The effects of stress, mood, and coping on blood glucose in NIDDM: A prospective pilot evaluation. Behav Res Ther 1994; 32:503–510.[31]

Study design: Multiple case study followed for 8 days.

Sample size: 8

Study population: Eight adults with non–insulin-dependent diabetes mellitus were identified through the outpatients of a university medical center. There were seven women and one man. They had no other medical diagnoses. They all were taking oral hyperglycemic agents.

Outcomes: Blood glucose measured on awakening and 2 hours after each meal. Subjective stress (SUDS) was rated on a scale of 0 (no stress) to 10 (extreme stress). Six Moods (sad, happy, anxious, angry, comfortable, and calm) also were rated on a 0 (none) to 10 (very much) scale. SUDS and Moods were measured immediately before each blood glucose determination. The DSI, a 58-item inventory of daily stresses, was completed each night and scored to obtain a stress measure. Exercise level was measured using a pedometer. A diet of equivalent energy value was used on days 1, 3, 5, and 7 and on days 2, 4, 6, and 8.

Comparisons: Differences between mean blood glucose values on high-stress and low-stress days were the main outcomes.

The Evidence

Comparison	High DSI Stress Days	Low DSI Stress Days	P Value
Mean blood glucose	210 mg/dL	189 mg/dL	<0.03
Mean blood glucose when exercise (pedometer reading) controlled for	208 mg/dL	192 mg/dL	NS

Comparison	High SUDS Stress Days	Low SUDS Stress Days	P Value
Mean blood glucose	208 mg/dL	185 mg/dL	<0.01
Mean blood glucose when exercise (pedometer reading) controlled for	206 mg/dL	187 mg/dL	NS

NS, not significant.

Interpretation: This small study shows an interesting relationship between daily blood glucose measurements and daily stress levels. Blood glucose was about 10% higher on high-stress days. Exercise levels were lower on high-stress days, and this could account for the higher blood glucose measurements.

In another study of the effect of stress on glycemic control in 55 adults with insulin-dependent diabetes, Lloyd et al[64] also found a relationship between hemoglobin A_{1c} levels and stress levels of the previous month.

Bottom line: In patients with non–insulin-dependent diabetes mellitus, blood glucose levels may be higher on days of high stress. This effect could be due to lower activity on those days, so encouraging patients to exercise during times of stress may be helpful.

What did Dr. Sharpe do?

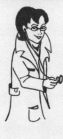

Dr. Sharpe told Mrs. Sampson that stress may lead to an increase in blood glucose. She advised her not to be too concerned about it at this point, to continue with her diet, and to try to get out for some exercise by walking. She did not adjust the oral hypoglycemic dosage at this point.

Reflection Exercise: How does this evidence apply to your practice? Would you apply this evidence to the management of appropriate patients in your practice? How will your practice change?

Joanne's Fear
(Pregnancy)

Nick and Joanne married 5 years ago just before you arrived in Bedford. You delivered their first child, Harry, 3 years ago. Joanne is now 12 weeks pregnant and was in for her first prenatal visit a month ago.

Her first delivery had been a difficult one. She had progressed to full dilation without any problems, but after 2 hours in the second stage of labor the fetus began to develop some serious drops in heart rate. A scalp gas value was not reassuring, so a cesarean section was advised and was done. Mom and baby did very well.

Joanne had decided she would like a trial of labor again this time to see if she can have a VBAC (vaginal birth after cesarean). She had a number of questions about it that you couldn't answer, so you promised to find the answers and let her know at her next visit. This is her next visit, but you know there is something else on her mind, recalling Cecilia's visit a few days ago and the headlines in the papers the past few days. The *Bedford Post:* NICK SAMPSON MISSING UNDER MYSTERIOUS CIRCUMSTANCES. The *Evening News:* BEDFORD MAN SUSPECT AFTER BODY FOUND.

Your nurse, after weighing her, checking her urine, and spending a little time talking with her, puts Joanne in your examining room. You touch Joanne on the shoulder as you enter and say you know she must be very worried. Looking very tired, probably in need of sleep, she says she is extremely worried and proceeds to tell you what has been happening.

Alex and Pierre had gone back to the airport parking garage early the morning after Nick hadn't returned home and found the car still there. Nick's luggage and fishing gear were in the back seat, not in the trunk. They had Joanne's spare keys to the car, so they opened the doors but found nothing to indicate where Nick might be. His luggage had been opened, but they couldn't tell if anything was missing. They then went to the trunk, which they had a little trouble opening. They wondered if it had been because someone had been playing with the lock to get into the trunk, but they saw no scratch marks to suggest this. When they finally got into the trunk, they found it stuffed with a large garbage bag. Their immediate thought was that it was a body, probably Nick's body. Alex stepped back from the truck feeling weak. Pierre opened the bag. It was a body—a woman's body, not Nick's. They called the police immediately.

The family had just received news this morning, in the form of a telephone call from the Toronto police. The woman in the trunk was Amy Stephens. No one in the family knows her. Joanne said she keeps feeling as if she knows the name from somewhere but can't remember. At least it wasn't Nick's body, she said. But where is Nick? Why hasn't he called? She is also worried because the police are now looking for him. Nick is their prime suspect in the murder.

You chat with Joanne for a while, empathizing with her and reassuring her that there are many possible explanations for this strange story and it will probably all be clear in a few days. After checking her blood pressure, which is normal, you check for a fetal heart. You find it, 140 beats/min and strong. It is the one happy moment in the visit, then Joanne starts to cry because Nick is not here to experience it with her. You chat with her a little longer until she settles. You think to yourself that Joanne will get through this however it turns out. She is from solid, stoic stock. Her father was a Baptist minister until he retired a few years ago. She was brought up with strong beliefs and taught to put her faith in God. She has admitted that she no longer holds the same depth of faith as her parents, but it is obvious to you that she has a strength to call on in times of trouble, whether it is hers or from a higher power.

You recall that her vaginal swabs came back from her last visit positive for *Gardnerella vaginalis*. You wonder if you should treat this or not, and, if so, should you use metronidazole? You also remember you should do a urine culture at this point in her pregnancy. So much to try to keep in mind. Fortunately she is coming back in a week. You thought it best that you see her a bit more frequently given the situation.

After she leaves, you realize the visit has taken a long time. But it couldn't be helped; some things just can't be rushed. But now you are 30 minutes behind. You head for examination room 2 still thinking about the clinical questions to which you need to find answers.

Some questions arising from this clinical encounter

4   In a 35-year-old woman, pregnant for the second time and after having had a cesarean section for her first infant 3 years previously, what is the likelihood of a successful outcome in a VBAC attempt for this pregnancy? What are the risks?

5   In a 35-year-old woman who is 12 weeks pregnant and has asymptomatic bacterial vaginosis, does antibiotic treatment have any effect on pregnancy outcome?

6   In a 35-year-old woman who is 12 weeks pregnant and has asymptomatic bacterial vaginosis, will treating the infection with metronidazole adversely affect the fetus?

7   In a 35-year-old woman who is 12 weeks pregnant and has asymptomatic bacteriuria, should the bacteria be eradicated with antibiotics?

Reflection Exercise:

What are your thoughts regarding these questions? Consider them in the context of your own practice. Consider what you might do before you read the evidence.

Citation: Mozurkewich EL, Hutton E. Elective repeat cesarian delivery versus trial of labor: A meta-analysis of the literature from 1989 to 1999. Am J Obstet Gynecol 2000; 183:1187–1197.[72]

Study design: Systematic review with meta-analysis.

Data sources: Cochrane Library, Medline, Embase, hand searching of references in articles. No attempt made to identify unpublished data.

Number of studies: 15

Number of patients: 47,682

Time frame: 1989–1999

Article selection criteria: Retrospective cohort and prospective cohort studies were included. No randomized controlled trials were identified. Studies were included if women in the elective repeat cesarean section (ERS) group had been considered eligible for a trial of labor (TOL) and if the study evaluated one or more of the outcomes of interest.

Data extraction: The outcomes of interest were uterine rupture, maternal mortality, fetal or neonatal mortality, 5-minute Apgar score <7, maternal febrile morbidity, maternal transfusion, and hysterectomy. Tests of heterogeneity were performed.

Article appraisal process: Data were extracted independently by both authors. Discrepancies were resolved by consensus. Studies were evaluated for quality and assigned a score.

Statistical heterogeneity tests? No.

Publication bias testing? No.

Other study details: Of the 28,813 women in the TOL arms of the studies, 20,746 achieved a successive virginal birth. The weighted average for this was 72.3% (95% confidence interval, 71.8–72.8%).

The Evidence

Outcome	EER (Trial of Labor)	CER (Elective Repeat Section)	Peto Odds Ratio	ARR	NNTh
Uterine rupture	77 of 17,613 (0.4%)	22 of 11,433 (0.2%)	2.1 (1.45–3.05)	0.2%	500
Maternal mortality	3 of 27,504 (0.01%)	0 of 11,433 (0)	1.52 (0.36–6.38)	NA	NA
Fetal or neonatal mortality	136 of 23,286 (0.6%)	56 of 16,239 (0.3%)	1.75 (1.30–2.28)	0.3%	333
5-Minute Apgar score < 7	41 of 1830 (2%)	14 of 1483 (0.9%)	2.24 (1.29–3.88)	1.1%	91

EER, experimental event rate; CER, control event rate; ARR, absolute risk reduction, NNTh, number needed to treat to harm 1 person; NA, not applicable as there is no significant difference.

The Evidence

Outcome	EER (Trial of Labor)	CER (Elective Repeat Section)	Peto Odds Ratio	ARR	NNTb
Maternal febrile morbidity	264 of 17,613 (1.5%)	262 of 11,433 (2.3%)	0.70 (0.64–0.77)	0.8%	125
Maternal transfusion required	100 of 8988 (1.1%)	94 of 5450 (1.8%)	0.57 (0.42–0.76)	0.7%	143
Hysterectomy	43 of 26,786 (0.16%)	71 of 17,337 (0.4%)	0.39 (0.26–0.56)	0.24%	416

EER, experimental event rate; CER, control event rate; ARR, absolute risk reduction; NNTb, number needed to treat to benefit 1 person.

Interpretation: It is important to note the direction of the effect in the two tables. In the first table, the odds ratios are >1, meaning the adverse outcome occurs more often in the TOL group. In the second table, odds ratios are <1, meaning the adverse outcomes occur less often in the TOL group.

Uterine rupture occurs more often in the TOL group. A total of 500 women would have to undergo a TOL to cause 1 more woman to have a ruptured uterus than would have occurred if a ERS had been done.

There was no significant difference in *maternal mortality* between the two groups, although three women died in the TOL group, and none died in the ERS group. Of the three women who died in the TOL group, two died of postoperative complications and the other died after aspiration of gastric contents at time of induction of anesthesia.

The newborns were more likely to have an *Apgar <7* in the TOL group. With every 91 trials of labor, there will be 1 newborn who will have an Apgar <7 who would not have had a low Apgar if an ERS had been carried out.

Maternal febrile morbidity was less in the TOL group. For every 125 ERS done, there will be 1 woman who will have maternal febrile morbidity that would not have occurred if a TOL had been done.

Maternal transfusion was required more often in the ERS group. For every 143 ERS done, there will be 1 woman who will require a transfusion who would not have required it if a TOL had been done.

Hysterectomy was more common in the ERS group. For every 416 ERS done, 1 woman will have a hysterectomy who would not have had one if a TOL had been done.

Bottom line: In women with a previous cesarean section, choosing to have a trial of labor in the subsequent pregnancy increases the likelihood of uterine rupture, fetal or neonatal death, and an Apgar of <7. It decreases the likelihood of maternal febrile morbidity, requirement for maternal blood transfusion, and requirement for a hysterectomy. The absolute risks and benefits are small, and the numbers needed to treat are large. It would be important to counsel patients of the risks and benefits of both options. Much weight should be given to the woman's preference because on balance one option is not much better or worse than the other.

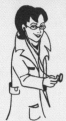

What did Dr. Sharpe do?

Dr. Sharpe reviewed the evidence with Joanne on her next visit. Joanne decided to try for a VBAC, recognizing the risks. The 72% likelihood of a successful VBAC, along with the rarity of serious outcomes even if a cesarean section were required, was what made the decision for her.

Reflection Exercise: How does this evidence apply to your practice? Would you apply this evidence to the management of appropriate patients in your practice? How will your practice change?

Answers to Questions 5 and 6

Preamble

We are dealing with these two questions together. Although we have asked only two questions in the scenario, there are three crucial questions to be answered in this situation:

1. Does having bacterial vaginosis (BV) predispose to adverse outcomes in pregnancy?
2. If so, does treating the BV decrease the likelihood of these adverse outcomes?
3. Is metronidazole safe to use during pregnancy?

We have found high-level evidence that answers these three questions.

Citation: Flynn CA, Helwig AL, Meurer LN. Bacterial vaginosis in pregnancy and the risk of prematurity: A meta-analysis. J Fam Pract 1999; 48:885–892.[27]

Study design: Systematic review with meta-analysis of case-control and cohort studies looking at the association of BV with selected pregnancy outcomes.

Data sources: Cochrane Library, Medline, and hand searching of references. Also contacted authors who had published on the subject in an attempt to identify unpublished data.

Number of studies: 19

Number of patients: 17,000

Time frame: 1984–1995

Article selection criteria: Case-control or cohort studies were included if they met the following criteria: (1) The study population was pregnant women; (2) the risk factor considered was the presence of BV; (3) the outcomes measured included either gestational age or birth weight; secondary outcomes considered were preterm (<37 weeks) delivery, preterm premature rupture of membranes, and preterm onset of labor.

Article appraisal process: Inclusion criteria and article assessment criteria were applied independently by the two investigators; differences were settled by consensus.

Data extraction: Data abstracted included country, medical setting, baseline risk of prematurity, inclusion and exclusion information, and method and timing of BV diagnosis.

Statistical heterogeneity tests? Yes. Homogeneity criteria were met for the outcomes of low birth weight, preterm premature rupture of membranes, and preterm onset of labor ($p > 0.33$ on heterogeneity test) but were not met for preterm delivery ($p < 0.05$ on heterogeneity test).

Publication bias testing? Yes. Authors were contacted to determine if unpublished data existed. A funnel plot was drawn, which did not suggest publication bias.

The Evidence

Outcome	EER (Pooled Event Rate for StudyGroup [BV Present])	CER (Pooled Event Rate for Comparison Group [No BV])	Peto Odds Ratio and 95% Confidence Interval	ARI	NNEh
Preterm delivery (< 37 wk)	472 of 3111 (0.151)	1349 of 14,167 (0.095)	1.85 (1.62–2.11)		18
Low birth weight (< 2500 g)	Unavailable	Unavailable	1.57 (1.32–1.87)	NA	NA
Preterm premature rupture of membranes*	82 of 699 (0.117)	359 of 3045 (0.117)	1.83 (1.39–2.44)	NA	NA
Premature onset of labor	178 of 574 (0.31)	658 of 2732 (0.24)	2.19 (1.73–2.76)	7%	14

EER, experimental event rate; BV, bacterial vaginosis; CER, control event rate; ARI, absolute risk increase; NNEh, number needed to be exposed to harm 1 person; NA, not applicable as there is no significant difference.

*Because of the weighting awarded the individual studies, the odds ratio is significant, but the absolute numbers used to calculate NNEh show no difference for this outcome.

Interpretation: Details of results were given only for preterm delivery in the article. We obtained detailed results from the authors for preterm premature rupture of membranes and preterm labor but not for low birth weight. The results available showed that BV increased the risks of all the outcomes, but we could calculate the number needed to be exposed to harm 1 person for only two. These results strongly suggest that the presence of BV in pregnant women increases the risk of all the outcomes considered.

Bottom line: Low birth weight, preterm (<37 weeks) delivery, preterm premature rupture of membranes, and preterm onset of labor all are increased by the presence of BV in pregnant women.

Citation: Brocklehurst P, Hannah M, McDonald H: Interventions for treating bacterial vaginosis in pregnancy. Cochrane review. In: The Cochrane Library, Issue 4. Oxford: Update Software; 2000.[11]

Study design: Systematic review with meta-analysis of randomized controlled trials looking at the effect of any antibiotic treatment for BV on selected pregnancy outcomes.

Data sources: Used standardized Cochrane Collaborative Review Group search strategy.

Number of studies: 5

Number of patients: 1504

Time frame: 1991–1997

Article selection criteria: All randomized controlled trials that compared (1) one antibiotic regimen with placebo or no treatment and (2) two or more alternative antibiotic regimens in pregnant women with BV. Women of any age at any stage of pregnancy with a diagnosis of BV regardless of method of diagnosis were included.

Article appraisal process: Data extraction and quality assessment were done independently by three reviewers.

Data extraction: Maternal and neonatal outcomes were considered and maternal side effects.

Statistical heterogeneity tests? Yes.

Publication bias testing? Not mentioned.

The Evidence

Outcome (in All Pregnant Women)	Pooled EER (Oral Antibiotic)	Pooled CER (Placebo or No Treatment)	Peto Odds Ratio and 95% Confidence Intervals	ARR	NNTb
Preterm premature rupture of membranes	14 of 473 (0.029)	26 of 464 (0.056)	0.48 (0.25–0.92)	2.7%	37
Preterm delivery (<37 wk)	93 of 645 (0.144)	90 of 550 (0.164)	0.61 (0.43–0.87)	2%	50
Preterm delivery (<34 wk)	9 of 286 (0.031)	10 of 274 (0.036)	0.83 (0.33–2.08)	NA	NA
Preterm delivery (<32 wk)	5 of 242 (0.021)	5 of 238 (0.021)	0.98 (0.28–3.44)	NA	NA
Low birth weight (however defined)	6 of 44 (0.136)	12 of 36 (0.333)	0.33 (0.11–0.93)	19.7%	5

EER, experimental event rate; CER, control event rate; ARR, absolute risk reduction; NNTb, number needed to treat to benefit 1 person; NA, not applicable as there is no significant difference.

The Evidence

Outcome (in Women With Previous Preterm Delivery)	Pooled EER (Antibiotic Treatment)	Pooled CER (Placebo or No Treatment)	Peto Odds Ratio and 95% Confidence Intervals	ARR	NNTb
Preterm premature rupture of membranes	3 of 66 (0.045)	15 of 60 (0.25)	0.18 (0.07–0.48)	20.5%	5
Preterm delivery (<37 wk)	57 of 187 (0.3)	58 of 116 (0.5)	0.37 (0.23–0.60)	20%	5
Preterm delivery (<34 wk)	4 of 61 (0.065)	7 of 53 (0.132)	0.49 (0.14–1.68)	NA	NA
Preterm delivery (<32 wk)	1 of 17 (0.058)	2 of 17 (0.117)	0.49 (0.05–5.08)	NA	NA
Low birth weight (however defined)	6 of 44 (0.136)	12 of 36 (0.333)	0.33 (0.11–0.93)	19.7%	5

EER, experimental event rate; CER, control event rate; ARR, absolute risk reduction; NNTb, number needed to treat to benefit 1 person; NA, not applicable as there is no significant difference.

Interpretation: In addition to the results in the tables, the studies looked at rates of neonatal sepsis, rates of uterine infections, and cure rate of BV. There was no difference in neonatal sepsis or uterine infections between patients treated and not treated in either all women or high-risk women. The cure rate with treatment (oral or vaginal) was about 75%. The authors of this Cochrane report concluded that the results do not support screening and treating all pregnant women for BV. They believed, however, that detection and treatment of women with a previous history of preterm birth may prevent a proportion of these women from having a further preterm birth.

When the results for all pregnant women (first table: low and high risk combined) are considered, it appears we would need to treat 37 women who have BV to prevent 1 from having a preterm premature rupture of membranes. Are the infants of these mothers who have preterm premature rupture of membranes faring any worse? They are more likely to deliver before 37 weeks but not before 34 weeks. Generally, infants born 34 weeks and after do okay. They are not more likely to get sepsis, but they are of lower weight as would be expected. It would seem that treating BV does make a difference, but that difference is probably of small consequence. It probably is not cost-effective to screen and treat everyone. If a physician already is doing this screening regularly now, however, there is not good evidence to recommend stopping it because it may be of some benefit.

What of women who have had a previous preterm delivery? The numbers are quite different here. It is only the preterm premature rupture of membranes, delivery <37 weeks, and low birth weight in which a difference was seen to be significant, but the size of the difference is much larger and the number needed to treat is only 5. The other consideration is that the sample sizes for delivery <34 weeks and <32 weeks were so small that it is highly probable that a large study would show a significant difference. Screening and treating women in this category is probably of benefit.

Bottom line: Pregnant women who have had a previous preterm delivery should be screened for BV and treated if the condition is present because treatment in this group substantially decreases preterm premature rupture of membranes, preterm delivery, and low-birth-weight infants. The evidence for screening and treating low-risk pregnant women is weak, however.

Citation: Carey JC, Klebanoff MA, Hauth JC, et al. Metronidazole to prevent pre-term delivery in pregnant women with symptomatic bacterial vaginosis. N Engl J Med 2000; 342:534–540.[14]

This study is being considered here because it was published after the Cochrane review reported previously and was not included in that review. It also deals specifically with asymptomatic BV, which is what the patient Joanne Walters-Sampson actually had.

Study design: Randomized controlled trial, double-blind, with intention-to-treat.

Sample size: 1953

Study population: Pregnant women, between 16 and 24 weeks' gestation, who were diagnosed with BV. Exclusion criteria included symptomatic vaginal discharge, had received antibiotics within the previous 2 weeks, and abused alcohol.

Intervention: (N = 953; 953 analyzed): Metronidazole, two 2-g dosages, 48 hours apart. The investigators quote a meta-analysis showing this regimen to be as effective as a 7-day regimen.

Control: (N = 966; 966 analyzed): A capsule with lactose was used for placebo. It looked the same as the capsule containing the metronidazole.

Outcomes: Preterm delivery, preterm premature rupture of membranes, and low birth weight.

The Evidence

Outcome	EER (Metronidazole)	CER (Placebo)	Relative Risk	ARR	NNTh
Preterm premature rupture of membranes	40 of 953 (4%)	36 of 966 (3%)	1.1 (0.7–1.8)	NA	NA
Preterm delivery (<37 wk)	116 of 953 (12.1%)	121 of 966 (12.5%)	1.0 (0.8–1.2)	NA	NA
Low birth weight (<2500 g)	103 of 953 (10.8%)	109 of 966 (11.3%)	1.0 (0.7–1.2)	NA	NA
Preterm delivery (<37 wk) in women with previous preterm delivery	24 of 80 (30%)	18 of 80 (22.5%)	1.3 (0.8–2.3)	NA	NA

EER, experimental event rate; CER, control event rate; ARR, absolute risk reduction; NNTh, number needed to treat to harm 1 person; NA, not applicable as there is no significant difference.

Interpretation: This fairly large randomized controlled trial shows no difference in either low-risk or high-risk groups for any of the outcomes measured. Whether or not the BV was treated made no difference to outcome. These results do not agree with the results found in the Cochrane systematic review. The sample size of this one study was also larger than the combined sample sizes of the studies included in the Cochrane review. It is often thought that a single, large, well-conducted randomized controlled trial is more reliable than a systematic review. To help us determine the correct answer, we used software available from the Cochrane website called RevMan and added the results of this new randomized controlled trial to the studies they had used in their systematic review. The results of this one study when added to the Cochrane review changed all of the outcomes to being nonsignificant in the pregnant women and high-risk women groups.

There are a few caveats. This study was only in asymptomatic women with BV. What about symptomatic women? A larger percentage of women in the metronidazole group had vomiting after they took the medication. This circumstance may have led to a lessened effect of the treatment. The investigators used a treatment regimen that, although more likely to achieve compliance with the full dose, may not be as effective at preventing the effects of BV on pregnancy as the usual 7-day regimen.

Bottom line: This large randomized controlled trial failed to show any effect of treating asymptomatic BV on the adverse effects known to be associated with the presence of BV in pregnant women.

Combined bottom line: The randomized controlled trial and a meta-analysis done by combining the results of this trial with an older meta-analysis strongly suggest that treatment of BV during pregnancy does not reduce the risk of preterm premature rupture of membranes, premature delivery, or low birth weight in either low-risk or high-risk pregnant patients. Because of some uncertainties about the treatment regimen in the recent randomized controlled trial, and because a meta-analysis that does not include this recent trial suggests that there may be benefit in patients with previous preterm deliveries, one could not fault physicians for continuing to treat BV, at least in high-risk patients. The balance of the evidence does suggest that it is not effective, however.

Citation: Burtin P, Taddio A, Ariburnu O, et al. Safety of metronidazole in pregnancy: A meta-analysis. Am J Obstet Gynecol 1995; 172:525–529.[13]

Study design: Systematic review with meta-analysis of articles reporting on metronidazole use in pregnancy.

Data sources: Medline, references in textbooks, hand searching of references of articles.

Number of studies: 7

Number of patients: 155,499

Time frame: 1964–1987

Article selection criteria: Articles were included if they compared women who used metronidazole during the first trimester of pregnancy with a group who either did not use metronidazole at all during pregnancy or used it only during the third trimester. Studies also had to have as the outcome the occurrence of birth defects in live-born infants. Studies were included only if they had at least 10 women who were exposed to metronidazole.

Article appraisal process: Two independent reviewers with nonmedical backgrounds reviewed each article for inclusion criteria.

Statistical heterogeneity tests? Yes. Studies were homogeneous, $p = 0.636$.

Publication bias testing? No, but discussed and thought unlikely.

Other study details: Not sufficient numbers to assess other outcomes, such as miscarriages and stillbirths. They did a sensitivity analysis, however, by assuming a worst-case scenario and added the two of these events (one miscarriage and one stillbirth) in these studies and still did not get a significant effect of metronidazole on outcomes.

The Evidence

Outcome	EER (Metronidazole Exposure First Trimester)	CER (No Metronidazole Exposure During First Trimester)	Odds Ratio and 95% Confidence Interval	ARR	NNTh
Birth defects	68 of 1336 (5.1%)	9859 of 154,163 (6.4%)	0.93 (0.73–1.18)	NA	NA

EER, experimental event rate; CER, control event rate; ARR, absolute risk reduction; NNTh, number needed to treat to harm 1 person; NA, not applicable as there is no significant difference.

Interpretation: This meta-analysis, which includes large numbers of patients, fairly convincingly shows that metronidazole is not harmful in the first trimester of pregnancy. When just the major malformations are looked at (e.g., anencephaly, microcephaly, hydrocephalus, clubfoot, harelip), 14 occurred in the control groups, and only 1 occurred in the metronidazole group.

Bottom line: Metronidazole taken during the first trimester of pregnancy does not increase the likelihood of birth defects.

Overall Bottom Line Answers to the Three Questions about BV in Pregnancy

1. Does having BV predispose to adverse outcomes in pregnancy? *Yes. Women with BV are more likely to have preterm delivery, low-birthweight infants, preterm premature rupture of membranes, and premature onset on labor.*

2. If so, does treating the BV decrease the likelihood of these adverse outcomes? *Probably not, but you still might consider treating in women who had a previous preterm delivery.*
3. Is metronidazole safe to use during pregnancy? *Yes, including in the first trimester.*

What did Dr. Sharpe do?

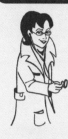

Dr. Sharpe wished that vaginal swab had never been taken! There was a tendency to want to treat the *Gardnerella* now that it had been detected. *Gardnerella* often is present in the vagina, however, without there being an infection. BV is more than just the presence of *G. vaginalis.* The study on asymptomatic BV was convincing. Although it would have been safe to give Joanne metronidazole, Dr. Sharpe decided not to treat and to begin a policy of not doing screening vaginal swabs on pregnant women except those who had a previous preterm delivery. The evidence suggested that even those women did not need to be screened, but there were a few questions about the study, so why take the chance.

Reflection Exercise: How does this evidence apply to your practice? Would you apply this evidence to the management of appropriate patients in your practice? How will your practice change?

Answer to Question 7

Citation: Smaill F. Antibiotics for symptomatic bacteriuria in pregnancy. Cochrane review. In: The Cochrane Library, Issue 4. Oxford: Update Software; 2000.[98]

Study design: Systematic review with meta-analysis.

Data sources: Cochrane Pregnancy and Childbirth Group trials register.

Number of studies: 13

Number of patients: 2465

Time frame: 1960–1987

Article selection criteria: Randomized trials comparing antibiotic treatment with placebo or no treatment in pregnant women with asymptomatic bacteriuria found on antenatal screening.

Article appraisal process: Single reviewer of articles.

Data extraction: Information was extracted on method of allocation, characteristics of participants, and type of interventions and outcomes.

Statistical heterogeneity tests? Yes. Studies were statistically similar.

Publication bias testing? Not mentioned.

The Evidence

Outcome	EER (Antibiotic Treatment)	CER (No Treatment)	Peto Odds Ratio	ARR	NNTb
Persistent bacteriuria	35 of 205 (17%)	176 of 210 (84%)	0.07 (0.05–0.10)	67%	1.5
Development of pyelonephritis	56 of 1037 (5.4%)	186 of 974 (19.1%)	0.25 (0.19–0.32)	13.7%	7
Preterm delivery or low birth weight	101 of 1044 (9.6%)	127 of 879 (14.4%)	0.60 (0.45–0.80)	4.8%	21

EER, experimental event rate; CER, control event rate; ARR, absolute risk reduction; NNTb, number needed to treat to benefit 1 person.

The Evidence

Outcome	EER (Short-Course [3–7 days] Antibiotics)	CER (No Treatment)	Peto Odds Ratio	ARR	NNTb
Persistent bacteriuria	9 of 37 (24.3%)	26 of 32 (81.2%)	0.11 (0.04–0.27)	56.9%	1.7
Development of pyelonephritis	19 of 359 (5.3%)	50 of 366 (14.5%)	0.35 (0.21–0.58)	9.2%	11
Preterm delivery or low birth weight	25 of 355 (7%)	48 of 300 (16%)	0.41 (0.25–0.67)	9%	11

EER, experimental event rate; CER, control event rate; ARR, absolute risk reduction; NNTb, number needed to treat to benefit 1 person.

Interpretation: Antibiotic effectively clears asymptomatic bacteriuria. In doing so, it decreases the likelihood of the woman developing pyelonephritis by about 14% and decreases the risk of preterm delivery by 5%. Short-course antibiotics, given for 3–7 days, seem to work as well as longer course antibiotics. The reduction in risk of preterm delivery was greater with short-term antibiotics.

The Cochrane Library also has a review that looks at the use of single-dose antibiotics for asymptomatic bacteriuria. There are few good trials, however, and this treatment has not been shown to be effective in decreasing the outcomes listed in the tables.

A meta-analysis done in 1989 by Romero et al[88] looked at women with untreated asymptomatic bacteriuria and women without bacteriuria. They found that women with asymptomatic bacteriuria were more likely to deliver preterm and to have low-birth-weight infants. They also looked at trials that compared treatment with no treatment of asymptomatic bacteriuria and found similar results as this Cochrane review.

Bottom line: Asymptomatic bacteriuria should be screened for and treated in early pregnancy. It decreases the risk of pyelonephritis, preterm delivery, and low-birth-weight infants.

What did Dr. Sharpe do?

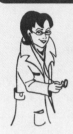

Dr. Sharpe plans to do a urine culture on the next visit. If it is positive, she plans to treat with an appropriate antibiotic. What is the appropriate antibiotic to use at this point in pregnancy? That's another question!

Reflection Exercise: How does this evidence apply to your practice? Would you apply this evidence to the management of appropriate patients in your practice? How will your practice change?

Alexander's Secret
(Hypertension)

When you first came to Bedford 5 years ago, Alexander Sampson came in with his wife Cecilia requesting that you take over their medical care. They had been patients of Dr. McCallum, your predecessor, who had left for greener pastures in the United States. Alex at that time was on hydrochlorothiazide, 50 mg daily, for hypertension. You subsequently decreased the hydrochlorothiazide to 25 mg daily after he lost 15 lb and his blood pressure remained controlled on the lower dosage. He also was able to stop the 3 potassium (Slow-K) tablets per day when the hydrochlorothiazide dosage was decreased. He has regained 10 lb, and his blood pressure was increased on the last visit. If it is increased again today, you likely will have to try to decrease it with medications. You are wondering if you should increase the hydrochlorothiazide to 50 mg or try something else.

You also note that you put him on atorvastatin, 10 mg, 3 months ago because his cholesterol was 7.3 mmol/L with a cholesterol-to-high-density lipoprotein (HDL) ratio of 6. You must remember to recheck his lipids and his liver enzymes.

You also recall that Alex started smoking again last year after stopping for 5 years. With his weight, his blood pressure, his cholesterol, and his smoking, you are worried he is setting himself up for a major cardiovascular event. He does not have a strong family history of heart disease or stroke. He denies any chest pain or symptoms of intermittent claudication or transient ischemic attacks. He had never had a myocardial infarction. But now with all this added stress!

Alex is indeed under a lot of stress. He asks if you have heard about his family's awful circumstance in the papers, and you tell him you have. He tells you about the trip he and Pierre made to Toronto. The story he tells doesn't differ substantially from what Joanne had told you except for the part about the argument he and Pierre had. Alex got upset with Pierre for "just taking off" out of the parking lot without waiting for Nick. He told Pierre that if he had waited perhaps none of this would have happened. You get the impression that Alex doesn't really like Pierre much.

Alex hadn't recognized the body when they found it in the trunk but knew immediately who it was when he heard the name from the police. But he hasn't told anyone, not the police or anyone in his family. It was a secret he shared with Nick. He is telling you now because he has to talk to someone about it, or it will gnaw at him until he can't stand it any more. He knows that you will keep it in confidence.

About 10 years ago, long before Nick and Joanne were married and even before they were dating, Nick had met Amy Stephens at a university bar. It was the end of term and the end of university for Nick, who was graduating from law school at the University of Toronto. Everyone was celebrating. Nick had more than usual to drink and ended up sleeping with Amy that night. She became pregnant, claimed it was Nick's, and threatened to have the child and take him to court if he didn't support her financially. The other option was for him to pay her a lump sum of $25,000, and she would have an abortion. It was blackmail, Nick realized, but to have this millstone around his neck at the beginning of his career was too much. He talked with his father about it, and Alex agreed to pay Amy the $25,000 with the understanding that Nick would pay it back over time.

At the time, Alex was very upset with Nick and with "this woman," but he agreed with Nick that it was best to give in to her demands and be done with it. Now she shows up dead in the trunk of Nick's car. It seemed that there must be some connection, but what? Had she approached Nick again and he killed her? It just didn't seem like him. Was it a coincidence that the body showed up in Nick's car? Someone with the keys must have put it there. Only Nick and Joanne had keys as far as he knew. But Joanne knew nothing about the past relationship between Nick and Amy. If Joanne had found out somehow, would she have been so upset as to kill Amy? That just didn't seem like Joanne either! But as far as Alex knew, only he and Nick and Amy knew about their little secret from 10 years past. Perhaps Amy told someone else. If she had told someone else, and if that person had killed her for some other reason, they might have tried to set Nick up by placing the body in his car. It would have had to be someone who knew Nick's car and knew it was at the airport parking garage.

It was all very confusing for Alex. He was going over and over it in his mind. He was a lawyer, but when something like this happens in your own family, it becomes difficult to know what to think. He just could not believe Nick was a murderer. He knew if he told the police about Amy's blackmail and the pay-off, they would charge Nick as soon as they found him. They had asked the whole family if anyone knew of any connection between Nick and the dead woman. Everyone had denied knowing her or any connection between her and Nick. Alex had denied it as well. One thing was true: He hadn't ever seen her before he saw her dead.

You spend the next 15 minutes chatting with Mr. Sampson. You don't have any more answers than he does. You are understanding and tell him that he has to make up his own mind about what to do with the information he has. You tell him he can feel assured his secret is safe with you, but you are feeling very uncomfortable.

You check Alex's blood pressure. It is 160/105 mm Hg, increased from 145/95 mm Hg at his last visit. You tell him you won't change his medications during such a time of stress because the elevated reading may be due to this current situation, but again you are not certain. Perhaps you should be treating him more vigorously. You give him a requisition to have fasting lipids and liver enzymes done. You think about telling him to stop smoking yet again but think better of it. He is unlikely to quit during this upheaval in his life, you think.

Some questions arising from this clinical encounter

8 In a 60-year-old man with uncontrolled hypertension on hydrochloro-thiazide, 25 mg daily, would increasing the dosage to 50 mg be likely to control his blood pressure? Would hypokalemia be an issue?

9 In a 60-year-old man with hyperlipidemia who was started on treat-ment with a statin drug just 3 months ago, how often should his lipids and liver enzymes be checked?

10 In a 60-year-old man with four risk factors for cardiovascular disease (overweight, hypertension, hyperlipidemia, and smoking), what is his risk of having a cardiovascular event over the next 5 years? (*Cardiovas-cular event* refers to the development of ischemic heart disease, pe-ripheral vascular disease, or cerebrovascular disease.)

11 Would Mr. Sampson benefit from ramipril according to the HOPE trial? If so, how much should he be taking?

12 A 60-year-old man with poorly controlled hypertension on medica-tion has a blood pressure measurement that is higher than his usually slightly elevated reading. What is the likelihood that this acute eleva-tion is due to a recent stress event in his life and should not be con-sidered when making a decision about treatment?

13 Is counseling to quit smoking effective during high stress points in a smoker's life?

Reflection Exercise:

What are your thoughts regarding these questions? Consider them in the context of your own practice. Consider what you might do before you read the evidence.

Answer to Question 8

Citation: Wright JM, Lee CH, Chambers GK. Systematic review of antihypertensive thera-pies: Does the evidence assist in choosing a first-line drug? Can Med Assoc J 1999; 161:25–32.[112]

Study design: Systematic review with meta-analysis.

Data sources: Medline, Cochrane Library, Embase, hand searching of references of previous reviews.

Number of studies: 23

Number of patients: 50,853

Time frame: 1966–1997

Article selection criteria: Randomized controlled trials of at least 1 year's duration that provided morbidity or mortality data and that compared one of six possible first-line antihypertensive therapies either with another one of the six drug therapies or with no treatment, including placebo. The six possible first-line therapies were thiazides, β-blockers, angiotensin-converting enzyme (ACE) inhibitors, calcium channel blockers (CCBs), α-adrenergic blockers, and angiotensin II receptor antagonists.

Article appraisal process: Two independent reviewers.

Data extraction: Patient demographics and outcomes.

Statistical heterogeneity tests? No.

Publication bias testing? No.

Other study details: The range for time of follow-up was 1–10 years with most trials being 2–6 years.

The Evidence

Outcome	EER (Low-Dose Thiazide [< 50 mg Hydrochlorothiazide Daily or Equivalent])	CER (No Treatment)	Relative Risk	ARR	NNTb
Death	521 of 4349 (12%)	720 of 5163 (13.9%)	0.89 (0.81–0.99)	1.9%	53
Stroke	197 of 4349 (4.5%)	355 of 5163 (6.9%)	0.66 (0.56–0.79)	2.4%	44
Coronary artery disease	221 of 4349 (5.1%)	374 of 5163 (7.2%)	0.71 (0.60–0.84)	2.1%	48
All cardiovascular events	527 of 4349 (12.1%)	899 of 5163 (17.4%)	0.68 (0.62–0.75)	5.3	19

EER, experimental event rate; CER, control event rate; ARR, absolute risk reduction; NNTb, number needed to treat to benefit 1 person.

The Evidence

Outcome	EER (High-Dose Thiazide [Equivalent to 50 mg Hydrochlorothiazide Daily or More])	CER (No Treatment)	Relative Risk	ARR	NNTb
Death	221 of 7769 (2.8%)	377 of 12,070 (3.1%)	0.90 (0.76–1.05)	NA	NA
Stroke	87 of 7769 (1.1%)	229 of 12,070 (1.9%)	0.47 (0.37–0.61)	0.8%	125
Coronary artery disease	212 of 7769 (2.7%)	329 of 12,070 (2.7%)	1.00 (0.84–1.19)	NA	NA
All cardiovascular events	311 of 7769 (4.0%)	613 of 12,070 (5.1%)	1.1%	0.72 (0.63–0.82)	91

EER, experimental event rate; CER, control event rate; ARR, absolute risk reduction; NNTb, number needed to treat to benefit 1 person; NA, not applicable as there is no significant difference.

Other results from this meta-analysis: In the two trials comparing β-blockers with placebo, β-blockers were no better than placebo in decreasing any of the outcomes.

In the one trial comparing CCBs with placebo, CCBs decreased stroke and total cardiovascular events but not death or coronary artery disease.

Thiazides lowered systolic blood pressure better than β-blockers or CCBs but were the same as β-blockers and CCBs for lowering diastolic pressure.

Low-dose and high-dose thiazides were about equally effective at lowering blood pressure. They both were better than β-blockers and CCBs at lowering systolic blood pressure.

In trials that compared thiazides with β-blockers directly, there were no differences in any of the outcomes, but there were significantly fewer side effects with thiazides.

No trials included in this review compared ACE inhibitors with placebo and looked at death and cardiovascular outcomes. There also were no trials that compared ACE inhibitors with thiazides.

Interpretation: Thiazides seem to be better than β-blockers and CCBs at decreasing blood pressure and at improving outcomes. When low-dose thiazides are compared with high-dose thiazides, the low-dose thiazides are better at preventing death, stroke, coronary artery disease, and total cardiovascular mortality than high-dose thiazides. This systematic review does not address the value of ACE inhibitors well, especially considering more recent evidence that ACE inhibition can have a marked effect on reducing cardiovascular events. The rate of hypokalemia in trials looking at low-dose thiazides has been low, about 1%, whereas rates of 30% have been reported for thiazides when higher does are used.

Bottom line: Low-dose thiazides decrease cardiovascular risk more than high-dose thiazides and lower blood pressure equally well.

What did Dr. Sharpe do?

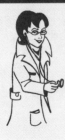

Dr. Sharpe did not increase Mr. Sampson's hydrochlorothiazide to 50 mg because the evidence suggests it would be of no benefit. He probably also would have had problems with hypokalemia. What to do? Should Dr. Sharpe stop the hydrochlorothiazide and start a different drug or keep him on low-dose hydrochlorothiazide and add another drug? If so, which drug? So many questions!

Reflection Exercise: How does this evidence apply to your practice? Would you apply this evidence to the management of appropriate patients in your practice? How will your practice change?

Preamble

This question was more difficult to answer than we expected. If you look at the monographs of the various statins, they all say approximately the same thing: The incidence of elevated hepatic enzymes in patients on their drug is around 1–2%. (We are using the term *statin* for all the hydroxymethylglu-taryl–coenzyme A reductase inhibitors.) The monographs also give approximately the same recommendations for monitoring:

1. Perform liver function tests before starting therapy.
2. Recheck at 12 weeks, then periodically indefinitely. Or check every 6 months for the first year of treatment or until 1 year after the last elevation in dose.
3. Patients who develop increased transaminase levels should be monitored with a second liver function evaluation to confirm the findings and be followed thereafter with frequent liver function tests until the abnormalities return to normal. Should an increase in aspartate aminotransferase (AST) or alanine aminotransferase (ALT) become more than three times the upper level of normal, statin therapy should be withdrawn.

One would think that these recommendations are based on fairly clear evidence linking statins with the elevation in liver enzymes or linking them with liver damage. It seems, however, that the abnormalities return to normal when the drug is stopped, and there has been no definite case of hepatitis that has been linked causally with these drugs.

These recommendations seem to be aimed at preventing litigation. We should look at the evidence as best we can, however. We were unable to find a study designed to look specifically at the effect of statins on the liver. Most of the large trials looking at the effect of statins on cardiovascular morbidity and mortality also report on biochemical abnormalities associated with the drugs. The following table reports on the data from two different trials.

The Evidence

Statin and Trial Name	EER (Elevated ALT [>3 times ULN] with the Statin)	CER (Elevated ALT [>3 times ULN] with Placebo)	Relative Risk	ARI	NNTh
Simvastatin 4S Trial[57]	49 of 2221 (2.2%)	33 of 2223 (1.5%)	1.47 (0.95–2.3)	NA	NA
Pravastatin West of Scotland Trial[58]	16 of 3302 (0.5%)	12 of 3293 (0.4%)	1.39 (0.65–2.9)	NA	NA

EER, experimental event rate; ULN, upper limits of normal; CER, control event rate; ARR, absolute risk reduction; NNTb, number needed to treat to benefit 1 person; NA, not applicable as there is no significant difference.

The Evidence

Statin and Trial Name	EER (Elevated AST [>3 times ULN] with the Statin)	CER (Elevated AST [>3 times ULN] with Placebo)	Relative Risk	ARI	NNTb
Simvastatin 4S Trial[57]	20 of 2221 (0.9%)	23 of 2223 (1%)	0.9 (0.5–1.6)	NA	NA
Pravastatin West of Scotland Trial[58]	26 of 3302 (0.8%)	20 of 3293 (0.6%)	1.3 (0.7–2.4)	NA	NA

EER, experimental event rate; ULN, upper limits of normal; CER, control event rate; ARR, absolute risk reduction; NNTb, number needed to treat to benefit 1 person; NA, not applicable as there is no significant difference.

Interpretation: The numbers from these two trials are representative of the low rates of liver enzyme irregularities that occur with statins. It probably would take an unusually large trial to show any significant difference, then the absolute risk increase would be so small as to be inconsequential. These two trials do not use atorvastatin, but the numbers are similar for all statins. Cases of rhabdomyolysis in patients using statins have increased concern about these drugs, however. Cerivastatin (Baycol) has been removed from the market. The risk of this condition with the other statins is extremely low. Still, if biochemical follow-up is going to be done, it might be prudent to include creatine kinase levels in the list.

What did Dr. Sharpe do?

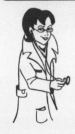

Being no fool, Dr. Sharpe decided to monitor Mr. Sampson and all patients on statins according to the pharmaceutical guidelines. Until professional organizations that produce clinical practice guidelines and set a standard for practice say whether or not it is necessary to do such ongoing monitoring, this is probably the best approach.

Reflection Exercise: How does this evidence apply to your practice? Would you apply this evidence to the management of appropriate patients in your practice? How will your practice change?

Preamble

Many schemes have been developed to assess the risk of cardiovascular disease in an individual patient. A good approach is used in the prediction guide developed for the National Heart Foundation of New Zealand by Jackson (Fig. 1). Using a color-coded scheme for risk levels, this guide assesses risk based on sex, age, blood pressure, cholesterol level, smoking status, and absence or presence of diabetes. The evidence for this prediction guide was reviewed and updated in the *British Medical Journal.*[48] The guide predicts the probability of occurrence of a cardiovascular event within the next 5 years. *Cardiovascular event* is defined as death related to coronary disease, nonfatal myocardial infarction, new angina, fatal or nonfatal stroke or transient ischemic attack, or the development of congestive heart failure or peripheral vascular disease.

What did Dr. Sharpe do?

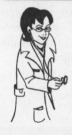

Dr. Sharpe used the chart to assess Mr. Sampson's risk of having a cardiovascular event in the next 5 years. He is male, age 60, a smoker, no diabetes, blood pressure is 160/105 mm Hg, and total cholesterol-to-HDL ratio is 6. Dr. Sharpe applied these data to the guide and determined that Mr. Sampson has a 25–30% probability of having a cardiovascular event in the next 5 years. This is high; the number needed to treat for benefit is only 11. This discovery redoubled Dr. Sharpe's determination to intensify her therapeutic efforts toward Mr. Sampson to decrease his risk. She calculated, using the guide again, that if she can control his blood pressure (<140.90 mm Hg) and lower his total cholesterol-to-HDL ratio to <5, she can decrease his risk to 15–20%. If he can stop smoking, his risk would be decreased further to 5–10%.

Reflection Exercise: How does this evidence apply to your practice? Would you apply this evidence to the management of appropriate patients in your practice? How will your practice change?

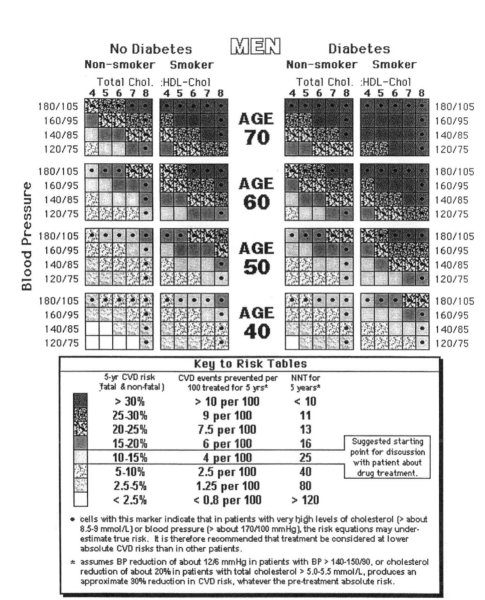

Fig. 1. Guides to assess risk of cardiovascular disease. (Reproduced with permission of the National Heart Foundation of New Zealand.) (*continued*)

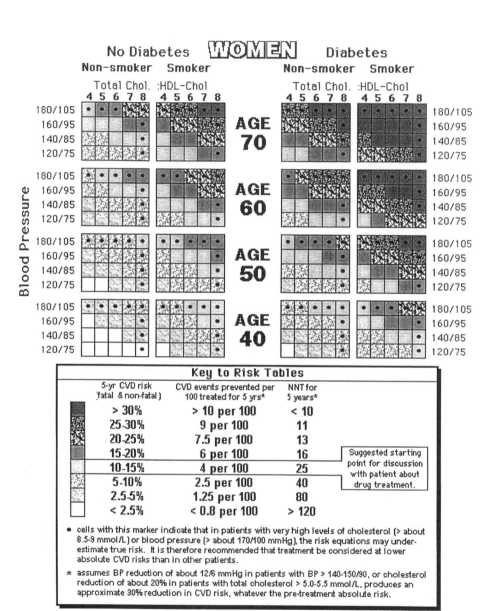

Fig. 1. (*Continued*)

Citation: The Heart Outcomes Prevention Evaluation Study Investigators. Effects of an angiotension converting enzyme inhibitor, ramipril, on cardiovascular events in high-risk patients. N Engl J Med 2000; 342:145–153.[102]

Study design: Randomized controlled trial, blinded, multicentered, with intention-to-treat analysis.

Sample size: 9297

Study population: Patients were recruited between 1993 and 1995 at 129 centers in Canada, 27 centers in the United States, 76 centers in 14 western European countries, 30 centers in Argentina and Brazil, and 5 centers in Mexico. Patients were eligible for the study if they were at least 55 years old; had a history of coronary heart disease, stroke, peripheral vascular disease, or diabetes; and had one other cardiovascular risk factor (hypertension, high cholesterol, cigarette smoking, or documented microalbuminuria). At baseline, the mean age was 66 years and 73.3% were men.

Intervention group: (N = 4645; 4645 analyzed): Ramipril, 10 mg once daily.

Control group: (N = 4652; 4652 analyzed): Placebo.

Outcomes: The main outcome was a composite of myocardial infarction, stroke, or death from cardiovascular disease. Secondary outcomes were death from any cause, need for revascularization, hospitalization for unstable angina or heart failure, and complications related to diabetes.

Other study details: Follow-up was 5 years.

The Evidence

Outcome	EER (Ramipril, 10 mg)	CER (Placebo)	Relative Risk	ARR	NNTb
Composite of myocardial infarction, stroke, or death from cardiovascular disease	651 of 4645 (0.14)	826 of 4652 (0.178)	0.78 (0.70–0.86)	3.8%	26
Death from noncardiovascular causes	200 of 4645 (0.043)	192 of 4652 (0.041)	1.03 (0.85–1.26)	NA	NA
Death from any cause	482 of 4645 (0.104)	569 of 4652 (0.122)	0.84 (0.75–0.95)	1.8%	56
Revascularization	742 of 4645 (0.16)	852 of 4652 (0.183)	0.85 (0.77–0.94)	2.3%	43
Hospitalization for unstable angina	554 of 4654 (0.119)	565 of 4652 (0.121)	0.98 (0.87–1.10)	NA	NA
Complications related to diabetes	299 of 4645 (0.064)	354 of 4652 (0.076)	0.84 (0.72–0.98)	1.3%	77
Heart failure	427 of 4645 (0.09)	535 of 4652 (0.115)	0.77 (0.67–0.87)	2.5%	40
Worsening angina	1107 of 4645 (0.238)	1220 of 4652 (0.262)	0.89 (0.82–0.96)	2.4%	42

EER, experimental event rate; CER, control event rate; ARR, absolute risk reduction; NNTb, number needed to treat to benefit 1 person; NA, not applicable as there is no significant difference.

Interpretation: Ramipril prevents death and several adverse cardiovascular outcomes in patients with established cardiovascular disease or diabetes. This effect is present even in patients without congestive heart failure or hypertension, meaning that the effect is not simply due to improvement in these conditions.

Bottom line: In patients with established cardiovascular disease or diabetes, the addition of ramipril to their therapeutic regimen decreases the likelihood of death, need for revascularization, heart failure, and worsening angina.

What did Dr. Sharpe do?

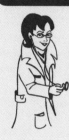

Mr. Sampson does not have established cardiovascular disease or diabetes, so he is not a candidate for ramipril according to this study. Dr. Sharpe decided that if she eventually starts Mr. Sampson on an ACE inhibitor, she will choose ramipril. It is possible that the effect shown with ramipril is a class effect and not limited to ramipril. Until the class effect has been established, however, she will use ramipril.

Reflection Exercise: How does this evidence apply to your practice? Would you apply this evidence to the management of appropriate patients in your practice? How will your practice change?

Answer to Question 12

Preamble

Rozanski et al[89] in a 1993 review of the literature concluded that there was clear and convincing evidence that psychological factors contribute significantly to the pathogenesis and expression of coronary artery disease. They also reported on 14 trials that looked at the effect of interventions designed to reduce stress on various cardiac end points. Four of the 14 trials resulted in a significant reduction in cardiac events. The trials usually were small, and they were so heterogeneous in outcome and intervention that a meta-analysis could not be done. We look at three studies that address the effect of stress and hypertension.

1. Baker et al[8] in 2000 reported that marital adjustment was one of the factors associated with left ventricular mass over 3 years in patients with mild hypertension.

2. In 1999, Spence et al,[100] in a major review of the evidence, found four major meta-analyses of the effect of stress management on hypertension. They recommended that for patients in whom stress seems to be an important issue, stress management should be considered as an intervention.

3. In a study that addresses more directly our question as it relates to Mr. Sampson, Vrijkotte et al[108] reported on the effects of work stress on ambulatory blood pressure. It is reviewed next.

Citation: Vrijkotte TGM, van Doornen LZP, de Geus EJC. Effects of work stress on ambulatory blood pressure, heart rate, and heart rate variability. Hypertension 2000; 35:880–886.[108]

Study participants: Middle-aged (35–55 years), white-collared workers performing mainly sedentary work, at a large computer company in Holland. Of the 820 who received a questionnaire, 460 (57%) responded. Of 460 participants, 300 agreed to participate, and of these, 187 who were in the upper and lower parts of the work stress scale were chosen.

Measurement scale: The Effort-Reward Imbalance questionnaire measures "effort" at work, which refers to the demanding aspects of the work environment, and "reward," which refers to esteem, monetary gratification, and status control. A high imbalance, with high effort but low reward, is considered high stress.

Outcome measures: 24-hour ambulatory monitoring.

Results: Participants classified as having a high imbalance had significantly higher work and home systolic blood pressure than participants not having high imbalance. This difference was on average 4 mm Hg. No difference was found for diastolic blood pressure. The increase in systolic blood pressure for high-imbalance individuals was greater at work than when they were at home, but the increased systolic blood pressure continued while at home even during leisure time.

Interpretation: Stress, defined as imbalance between work effort and work reward, has an effect on systolic blood pressure that continues throughout the day, not just while at work.

Bottom line: Given this and the other evidence, the effects of life stresses on measured blood pressure should be considered when making decisions about treatment adjustments in hypertensive patients. This is especially true for systolic blood pressure.

What did Dr. Sharpe do?

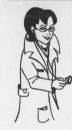

Dr. Sharpe decided to recheck Mr. Sampson before making changes to his medication. She was concerned about the current high-stress situation. She thought it was unlikely, however, that stress could account fully for an elevation to 160/105 mm Hg. So unless it decreased substantially, she planned to make a medication adjustment.

Reflection Exercise: How does this evidence apply to your practice? Would you apply this evidence to the management of appropriate patients in your practice? How will your practice change?

Comments: This is not an easy question. Parrott and Kaye[80] showed in a study of stress levels of smokers, nonsmokers, and abstaining smokers that if you deprive smokers of their "fix," they experience increased daily stress. Carey et al[15] looked at stress and smoking and concluded as others have that the relationship between the two is bi-directional. (1) Stress made it difficult to quit, (2) failure to quit causes stress, and (3) the process of quitting is stressful. From the balance of evidence, smokers would be less likely to be successful if they attempted to quit during a time of stress. We did not find a study that addresses this question directly, however.

What is needed is a study that rates smokers on their level of stress before smoking cessation counseling, then follows them to determine the proportion that are successful. We did not find such a study. Our hypothesis is that the success rate would be lower during time of stress.

What did Dr. Sharpe do?

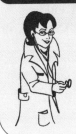

Dr. Sharpe was concerned about Mr. Sampson and knew she had to work on getting him to quit smoking. She decided, however, to wait until this whole murder affair has resolved somehow.

Reflection Exercise: How does this evidence apply to your practice? Would you apply this evidence to the management of appropriate patients in your practice? How will your practice change?

Nancy's Dilemma
(Oral Contraceptives)

Nancy Sampson-Savoy is the youngest child of Cecilia and Alexander Sampson. She married Pierre Savoy 2 years ago after becoming pregnant when a condom broke. They had been dating for about a year, although neither set of parents was happy with the relationship, especially Nancy's parents. It all seemed to have smoothed out after a year or so, judging by their comments when they came to see you for their various medical problems. The baby boy, Martin, who is now about 16 months old, certainly helped the situation. They all love him.

The delivery had gone well. Martin was born after just 4 hours of labor—8 lb, 7 oz and not even a tear. Physicians always take credit for lack of tears, but blame the infant's size or something else when there is one. In truth, it probably has little to do with the physician either way.

Nancy is in today because she is about to run out of oral contraceptive pills and needs a refill and her annual Pap smear. She also needed to get out of the house. She hasn't been at work since Nick disappeared. The whole family is trying to find him and trying to deal with all the terrible possibilities of what may have happened and where he may be right now. Cecilia is looking after Martin while Nancy is taking care of a few things today, including coming to see the doctor. That distasteful, necessary evil of the regular Pap smear!

You do the Pap smear and pelvic examination. You notice a little bit of an unusual discharge. You mention it to Nancy, who says she had noticed a little increase in discharge for over a month now but not much and it isn't itchy or foul-smelling. You send off vaginal and cervical swabs.

After the Pap smear, Nancy wants to talk. She says her parents are so distraught that she hasn't been able to sit down and discuss things with them properly, although she plans to tonight. Pierre seems to have got back to normal faster than anyone. He says he is letting the police do their job and not running off in all directions trying to find Nick like the Sampsons and Joanne are doing. Alex has even hired a private detective to try to find Nick. Nobody has heard anything yet. Nancy says she is glad Pierre is safe, but sometimes she thinks he knows more than he is letting on. It seems strange that Nick could disappear like that and Pierre know nothing about it. She tried to talk to him about it one evening after they had gone to bed, but perhaps she had used a blaming tone, because he got upset and just rolled over and went to sleep.

You are about to give her a refill for the pill when you realize she is on one of the newer ones with the third-generation progestin, desogestrel. You had read somewhere about these pills leading to a higher rate of deep vein thromboses. You give her the prescription but plan to check into it.

A question arising from this clinical encounter

14 In a 30-year-old woman with no risk factors, how much greater likelihood of developing deep venous thrombosis does she have with oral contraceptives containing desogestrel compared with oral contraceptives containing the earlier generation progestin, levonorgestrel?

Reflection Exercise:

What are your thoughts regarding this question? Consider this question in the context of your own practice. Consider what you might do before you read the evidence.

Answer to Question 14

Citation: Jick H, Kaye JA, Vasilakis-Scaramozza C, Jick SS. Risk of venous thromboembolism among users of third generation oral contraceptives compared with users of oral contraceptives with levonorgestrel before and after 1995: Cohort and case-control analysis. BMJ 2000; 321:1190–1195.[51]

Study design: Cohort and nested case-control analyses derived from the General Practice Research Database.

Sample size: Cohort: 1,340,776 (361,724 on levonorgestrel and 979,052 on desogestrel or gestodene)

Case-control: 675 (106 on oral contraceptives who had had venous thrombosis and 569 controls)

Study population: The General Practice Research Database provides information on personal characteristics, drugs prescribed, and clinical diagnoses for >3 million people, with follow-up as long as 12 years. In this study, there were two study periods, January 1993 to October 1995 and January 1996 to December 1999. Women in the study had to be on an oral contraceptive with desogestrel, gestodene, or levonorgestrel. Women who had venous thrombosis but with an obvious other cause were excluded (e.g., recent leg injury, recent surgery).

The Evidence: Cohort Study

Outcome	EER (Desogestrel or Gestodene)	CER (Levonorgestrel)	Relative Risk	ARI	NNTh
Venous thrombosis during study period 1 (1993–1995)	54 during 145,300 women-years at risk (0.00037)	17 during 83,600 women-years at risk (0.0002)	1.85	0.017%	5882
Venous thrombosis during study period 2 (1996–1999)	10 during 24,300 women-years at risk (0.00041)	25 during 108,100 women-years at risk (0.00023)	1.78	0.018%	5555

EER, experimental event rate; CER, control event rate; ARI, absolute risk increase; NNTh, number needed to treat to harm 1 person.

The Evidence: Case-Control Study

	Cases (with Venous Thrombosis) (n = 106)	Controls (without Venous Thrombosis) (n = 569)	Odds Ratio	NNTh
Desogestrel or gestodene	64	278	2.3	
Levonorgestrel	42	291	(1.3–3.9)	5500

NNTh, number needed to treat to harm 1 person.

Interpretation: It is important not to ignore evidence for harm by medications. It also is important not to overstate it. A balanced perspective is needed. The risk of venous thrombosis is approximately doubled with the third-generation oral contraceptives (desogestrel or gestodene) compared with the older oral contraceptives using levonorgestrel. The risk with the older oral contraceptives is only about 1 in 5000 women who take the pill for 1 year, however. With the newer pills, the risk is decreased to 1 in 3000. The number needed to treat is about 5500. This means a family physician would have to decide to put 5500 women on the older pill (levonorgestrel) instead of the newer pill (desogestrel) before 1 woman was prevented from having a venous thrombosis. Most family physicians would not prescribe the pill for that many women during their career. Other medications, such as nonsteroidal anti-inflammatory drugs (causing gastrointestinal bleeds) and benzodiazepines (causing falls), are much more likely to be harmful to patients.

The newer progestins double the rate, but it is two times a small number. The important issue is the awareness of the potential problem. Perhaps the newer progestins should be avoided in women with risk factors for venous thrombosis, such as a previous history or obesity. This study does not provide strong evidence for switching all patients who are doing fine on desogestrel or gestodene from that preparation to a preparation with levonorgestrel. A physician would have to switch 5500 patients before a benefit could be seen.

Bottom line: The newer oral contraceptives that use desogestrel or gestodene increase the risk of venous thrombosis by only a miniscule amount, 0.017%. Oral contraceptives should be considered contraindicated only in women who are at higher risk of venous thrombosis already. Women who are on the older pills and doing fine probably do not need to be switched. If the newer pills are better choice for a woman because of side-effect issues, they can be used with little risk. The woman should be informed, however, of the evidence in a balanced manner and involved in the decision.

What did Dr. Sharpe do?

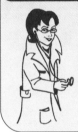

Dr. Sharpe kept Nancy on the newer pill. Nancy has no risk factors for venous thrombosis and has been having no side effects with the pill.

Reflection Exercise: How does this evidence apply to your practice? Would you apply this evidence to the management of appropriate patients in your practice? How will your practice change?

Pierre's Lie

(Ankle Injury)

You had met Pierre Savoy only on two other occasions—when he came in for a prenatal visit with Nancy, his wife, and again in the case room during the birth of their son, Martin. You never liked him much. He seemed slightly arrogant and didn't seem to treat Nancy very well. Nothing you could put a finger on, he just didn't do or say caring sorts of things when he was around her, the sort of things you have seen other men do in the same circumstance. Pierre had never been in to see you for any medical problem of his own, so you were surprised to see his name on your list this morning.

Pierre was complaining of an injured ankle. He said he had been in Toronto the day before and had stepped off a curb and rolled his foot over. He was able to walk on it, but it was painful when he walked. He felt it was worse today than yesterday. When you examined it, there was some swelling over the ankle, and it was a bit tender. You decided to send him for an x-ray. You had always found it difficult to know whether to x-ray injured ankles. They were almost always negative, but you didn't want to miss a fracture. You had heard something about some rules developed in Ottawa that you thought you would look up.

Pierre had gone to the hospital to get the x-ray done and came back to your office. You called the x-ray department and had Dr. O'Donnell, the radiologist, have a quick look at it for you. He said it looked fine, no evidence of fracture of the ankle. He noted, however, that the technician had x-rayed further up the leg than usual for an ankle injury because of a small laceration he had noticed high on the calf. There seemed to be some specks of metal as if a rusty nail had penetrated the leg. You embarrassingly thanked him. You realized you had not really had Pierre undress when you examined his ankle, just pulled up his pant legs a bit and had his shoe and sock off. That's generally enough for an ankle examination, but obviously not in this case. Just goes to show how important exposure and inspection is for the physical examination.

When you went back into the examining room, Pierre was gone. He had been in the adjacent room when you were speaking with Dr. O'Donnell. You wondered whether he wanted to avoid telling you how he had cut his leg. After lunch, you tried to reach him at his work but he wasn't in. Two days later, you received a copy of an emergency department (ED) note. Family physicians automatically received copies of ED notes in Bedford. Pierre had gone to the ED later the same day that you had seen him. He didn't mention to the ED physician that he already had seen his family physician. He told the ED physician that he had backed into a clean nail sticking out of the wall in his garage that afternoon. The ED physician cleaned it, irrigated it a little, and gave him a tetanus shot. This struck you as being strange. The x-ray technician had seen a cut in the morning, and the x-ray had shown old rust particles. Why was Pierre lying about what happened? Well, he would be back in to see you if that leg got infected! You would find out then.

Some questions arising from this clinical encounter

15 In a 35-year-old man with a history of an ankle injury, can the Ottawa ankle rules help determine the likelihood of a fracture and whether an x-ray should be done?

16 In a 35-year-old healthy man with a cellulitis in the calf from a puncture wound with a rusty nail, what is the most likely bacterium to be causing the infection, and what is the most appropriate antibiotic to use?

Reflection Exercise:

What are your thoughts regarding these questions? Consider them in the context of your own practice. Consider what you might do before you read the evidence.

Answer to Question 15

Citation: Auleley GR, Kerboull L, Durieux P, et al. Validation of the Ottawa Ankle Rules in France: A study in the surgical emergency department of teaching hospital. Ann Emerg Med 1998; 32:15–18.[5]

Study design: A prospective survey of patients.

Study population: Adults ≥18 years old who presented with acute ankle or mid-foot injury over a 4-month period to the ED of a teaching hospital in Paris.

Data: On each patient, the Ottawa ankle rules were applied, then the patient had an x-ray. The Ottawa ankle rules recommend that an x-ray be done if there is pain in the malleolar zone and inability to bear weight immediately and in the ED (4 steps) or there is bone tenderness at the posterior edge or tip of the malleolus.

The Evidence: Outcome of Ankle Injuries

	Fracture on X-Ray	No Fracture on X-Ray	Total
Ankle rules positive for fracture	48	171	219
Ankle rules negative for fracture	1	137	138
Total	49	308	357

Sensitivity = 98%; Specificity = 44%; positive predictive value = 22%; positive likelihood ratio = 176; negative likelihood ratio = 0.05; negative predictive value = 99%.

Interpretation: The Ottawa ankle rules is a SnNout; this means it is highly sensitive, and a negative test almost always rules out a fracture and an x-ray is unnecessary. If the test is positive, however, it is not specific enough to be certain that a fracture really does exist, and so an x-ray needs to be done to confirm the diagnosis.

Bottom line: The Ottawa ankle rules are useful, if negative, for ruling out an ankle fracture.

What did Dr. Sharpe do?

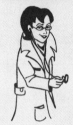

Pierre already had had an x-ray, and it was negative. Dr. Sharpe decided she would use the Ottawa ankle rules in the future to help decide whether or not to get an x-ray when someone presented with an ankle injury.

Reflection Exercise: How does this evidence apply to your practice? Would you apply this evidence to the management of appropriate patients in your practice? How will your practice change?

Answer to Question 16

Preamble

There are few data in the literature that directly address this question in adults. We found two relevant studies. Dupuy et al[24] addressed risk factors for leg cellulitis. They found that although factors such as leg ulcer, lymphedema, and toe intertrigo contribute the largest risk, a leg wound does increase the risk of developing cellulitis six times compared with developing cellulitis when no leg wound is present. The second study is of the causal organisms in cellulitis.

Citation: Hook EW, Hooton TM, Horton CA, et al. Microbiologic evaluation of cutaneous cellulitis in adults. Arch Intern Med 1986; 146:295–297.[45]

Study design: A microbiologic study of patients with cellulitis.

Study participants: Fifty patients seen in the ED at Harborview Medical Center, Seattle, who had a clinical diagnosis of cellulitis. Exclusion criteria were (1) age <16 years, (2) cellulitis involving head and neck, (3) history of antibiotic use in the previous week, (4) allergy to lidocaine, and (5) likelihood of another diagnosis (thrombophlebitis, abscess). There were 38 men and 112 women, age range from 23–84 years. Cellulitis was in the upper extremities in 4 patients and lower extremities in 46 patients.

Data collection: Four different cultures were taken. Primary lesion culture was done by swab when there was a defined break in the skin. Needle aspiration culture was done of the leading edge of the erythema. A punch biopsy culture was done at the leading edge of erythema. Blood cultures were taken.

Results: Thirteen (26%) patients had positive cultures. Twelve of the 13 cultures grew either streptococci or staphylococci. Seven of the 12 cultures grew both bacteria, 1 grew streptococci only, and 4 grew staphylococci only.

Interpretation: Several things are apparent. (1) Despite intensive culturing techniques, 74% of the cases of clinical cellulitis did not have positive cultures. (2) In the cases with positive cultures, *Staphylococcus aureus* was present in 85%. This would lead one to conclude that if antibiotics are to be prescribed, one that will be effective against *S. aureus* should be chosen.

Bottom line: Most cultures of cellulitis are negative. Cultures that are positive almost always grow *S. aureus*. An antibiotic effective against *S. aureus* should be used.

What did Dr. Sharpe do?

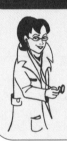

Based on this information, Dr. Sharpe concluded that Pierre was at a fairly high risk of developing cellulitis, and if he did, she would use cloxacillin to treat him.

Reflection Exercise: How does this evidence apply to your practice? Would you apply this evidence to the management of appropriate patients in your practice? How will your practice change?

Cecil Starkes
(Hematuria)

Mr. Starkes is a mildly obese man who quit smoking just last year after a severe bout of pneumonia nearly killed him. He has mild chronic obstructive pulmonary disease and hypertension. He is on salbutamol (Ventolin) and ipratropium bromide (Atrovent) inhalers twice daily and takes an angiotensin-converting enzyme inhibitor daily for his blood pressure.

Mr. Starkes is in today for a regular 3-month check. Your nurse dips his urine because he complained of some flank pain. There is a large amount of blood on the dipstick, and you see 10–20 red blood cells per high-power field when you check it using the microscope. There are a few white blood cells; the dipstick is negative for nitrates. He denies any symptoms of a urinary tract infection, and the back pain he referred to is classically musculoskeletal.

Examination of his back reveals no tenderness of the spine and no flank tenderness. His prostate is normal, as is examination of his penis and testicles. Abdominal examination is normal. You send him for a urine culture, which later comes back negative, as does a prostate-specific antigen test.

Some questions arising from this clinical encounter

17 In a 60-year-old man with asymptomatic hematuria and normal physical examination, what is the likelihood of significant pathology?

18 In a 60-year-old man with asymptomatic hematuria and normal physical examination, how useful is a renal and bladder ultrasound for ruling out significant disease?

Reflection Exercise:

What are your thoughts regarding these questions? Consider them in the context of your own practice. Consider what you might do before you read the evidence.

Preamble

We found two prospective studies[59,93] that investigated large cohorts of subjects with hematuria to determine outcome and best diagnostic approaches. One study comparing ultrasound and IVP also is considered.[73]

Citation: Murakami S, Igarashi T, Hara S, Shumazaki J. Strategies for asymptomatic microscopic hematuria: A prospective study of 1034 patients. J Urol 1990; 144:99–101.[73]

Study design: A prospective follow-up study of patients with asymptomatic microscopic hematuria.

Study population: Patients with asymptomatic microscopic hematuria on annual health examination who were referred to the urology clinic of a general hospital in Asahi City, Japan, between April 1982 and March 1987. Of the 1217 adult patients referred, 1034 were selected on the basis of >5 red blood cells/high-power field in the urine sediment on at least one of three urinalyses, urine protein ≤1+ on dipstick, and no history of urologic disorder. Average age of patients was 53.4 years. The male-to-female ratio was 1:3.

Investigations: Urine culture, urine cytology, coagulation studies, cystoscopy, ultrasonography, and excretory urography (IVP). Computed tomography and renal biopsy were performed in selected cases. In the case of insignificant lesions or when no cause was found, examinations were repeated every 6 months. In these cases, the average follow-up time as 3.8 years.

Categorization of findings: Highly significant lesions were those likely to be fatal without prompt treatment. With moderately significant lesions, the hematuria could be expected to resolve with treatment, but immediate treatment was not necessary because there was no threat to life. Insignificant lesions were those in which it was unclear whether they actually caused hematuria.

The Evidence: Outcomes After Initial Investigations on 1034 Patients

Highly significant lesions: 30 (2.9%)	Urologic malignancies	24
	Glomerulopathic conditions likely to progress to renal failure	6
Moderately significant lesions: 195 (18.9%)	Glomerulopathic conditions with preserved renal function	108
	Urinary calculi	50
	Urinary tract infection	18
	Hydronephrosis	10
	Caliceal diverticuli	3
	Vesicoureteral reflux	1
Insignificant lesions: 246 (23.8%)	Renal cyst	171
	Benign prostatic hypertrophy	31
	Chronic cystitis or other inflammatory changes in the bladder trigone seen on cystocopy	31
	Urethral caruncle	10
	Prostatic calculi	3
No lesions found: 563 (54.4%)		

The study also looked at the sensitivity and specificity of four of the tests used in the diagnosis. For this assessment, highly and moderately significant lesions were considered positive for disease, and insignificant lesions and no lesions were considered negative for disease.

Diagnostic Test	Sensitivity (%)	Specificity (%)
Urine culture	3.3	99.5
Cystoscopy	9.5	100
Ultrasound	24.5	99.2
Intravenous pyelography	54.5	99.6

Finally, the 809 people with insignificant or no lesions were followed every 6 months. After a mean follow-up of 3.8 years, 22 more lesions were found.

Renal calculi	9
Urinary tract infection	3
Glomerulonephritis	6
Bladder cancer	3
Prostatic cancer	1

Interpretation: Nearly 23% of adults presenting with asymptomatic hematuria have significant pathology. It is likely that this proportion is higher as age increases. Because the tests are highly specific but not very sensitive, a positive test rules in disease (few false-positives), but a negative test does not rule out disease. Patients with persistent hematuria and negative tests should be followed closely and probably should be referred to a urologist.

Bottom line: Asymptomatic hematuria is associated with a high likelihood of significant pathology. These patients should be investigated and followed closely if the cause of the hematuria is not apparent on initial investigations.

Citation: Khadra MH, Pickard RS, Charlton M, et al. A prospective analysis of 1,930 patients with hematuria to evaluate current diagnostic practice. J Urol 2000; 163:524–527.[54]

Study design: A prospective follow-up study of patients with asymptomatic microscopic and macroscopic hematuria.

Study population: Patients (1930) who attended a hematuria clinic at the Freeman Hospital in Newcastle-upon-Tyne, United Kingdom, between October 1994 and March 1997. Mean age was 58.3 years. There were 1194 men and 736 women.

Investigations: History and physical examination, "routine" blood tests, urinalysis, urine cytology, plain abdominal radiography, renal ultrasound, IVP, and flexible cystoscopy.

Follow-up: All patients were invited to return after 6 months for repeat midstream urine sampling and clinical assessment. Patients with no diagnosis on initial assessment continued to be monitored for subsequent development of significant causes of hematuria.

The Evidence: Summary of Diagnoses

Diagnosis	No. (%)
No diagnosis	1168 (60.5)
Renal cancer	12 (0.6)
Urothelial cancer	2 (0.1)
Bladder cancer	230 (11.9)
Prostate cancer	8 (0.4)
Stone disease	69 (3.6)
Urinary tract infection	251 (13)
Nephrologic disease	190 (9.8)

The likelihood of finding cancer for each gender and age group in the presence of microscopic and macroscopic hematuria is summarized in the next table.

The Evidence

| Age Group (y) | Females | | Males | |
	Microscopic Hematuria Percentage with cancer	Macroscopic Hematuria Percentage with cancer	Microscopic Hematuria Percentage with cancer	Macroscopic Hematuria Percentage with cancer
10–19	0	0	0	0
20–29	0	0	0	4.7%
30–39	0	0	1.7%	8.5%
40–49	2.9%	10.8%	1.3%	15.9%
50–59	1.9%	8.9%	1.9%	20.4%
60–69	4.5%	21.1%	7.9%	28.9%
70–79	4.5%	20.5%	17.4%	22.5%
80–89	15.8%	41.7%	21.1%	31.6%
90–99	0	33.3%	33.3%	50%

The 14 upper tract tumors were diagnosed using a combination of ultrasound and IVP. If ultrasound alone had been used, six tumors would have been missed; if IVP alone had been used, three tumors would have been missed. There were 230 patients with bladder cancer. Of these, only 60 showed a filling defect on IVP, and only 75 had positive urine cytology. Bladder ultrasound was not done in this study.

Interpretation: Although >60% of patients had no obvious reason for hematuria, nearly 40% had identified pathology, with 13% having cancer. The likelihood of cancer being present increases dramatically with age. Women >40 years old and men >30 years old should be investigated if they develop hematuria. Ultrasound and IVP are needed to rule out upper tract tumors (or alternately computed tomography scanning).

Bottom line: A large proportion of adults with hematuria have significant pathology and should be investigated. Upper tract disease can be ruled out with ultrasound and IVP, whereas diagnosis of lower tract disease requires urine culture and cystoscopy.

Overall conclusion: Asymptomatic hematuria should be investigated. The likelihood of significant pathology is 23–39%. The likelihood of a tumor being present is 3–13%. The likelihood increases with age and may be 20% in individuals >60 years old and 40% in individuals >80 years old. Ultrasound and IVP together can rule out most upper tract disease. Cystoscopy is needed to rule out bladder tumor. Because urothelial tumors are rare,[101] the order of the investigations might be ultrasound and cystoscopy first, and if the cause is not found and hematuria is persistent, then an IVP could be done.

What did Dr. Sharpe do?

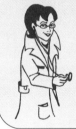

Dr. Sharpe ordered an ultrasound of kidney and bladder and arranged for Mr. Starkes to see a urologist.

Reflection Exercise: How does this evidence apply to your practice? Would you apply this evidence to the management of appropriate patients in your practice? How will your practice change?

INTERLUDE

The Bedford Family Medicine Clinic (BFMC) prided itself on being up-to-date. Its records were completely electronic, and the physicians practiced evidence-based medicine whenever possible. They allotted time each week to read and find answers to questions that had arisen in the course of practice. They were involved in teaching family medicine residents and medical students. The residents and students came from Queen's University in Kingston, a small city just 150 km from Bedford. The physicians had a teaching agreement with the Department of Family Medicine at Queen's.

The BFMC was a modern two-story building. The ground floor contained the physicians' offices, filing room, nurses' office, and reception/waiting area. Upstairs was a small staff lounge, a small library, and a storage area. The building, which backed onto a small lake, was across the street from the Bedford General Hospital. Larry and Janet Kelland lived across the lake from the clinic and sometimes came to work in their boat. Larry was one of the family physicians at the clinic, and Janet was a nutritionist at the hospital.

You and four other family physicians, two nurses, and two receptionists worked at the BFMC. Today was Wednesday, your CME afternoon, and you were on your way to Kingston to spend some time in the Bracken Library to find the answers to the many questions that had arisen over the past week or two. You enjoyed these educational times away from the practice. This was the best way to keep up-to-date. Going to the medical literature to find answers to real questions from real practice seemed to you to be the most useful type of continuing medical education.

But you had other things on your mind as you drove to Kingston. The call you had received from Nick Sampson was probably the most unusual thing that had happened to you in your 5 years of practice. You knew Nick and his wife Joanne fairly well. You had attended the birth of their child and remembered how wonderful Nick had been in supporting Joanne during labor. You also had been at several social functions with them, but you wouldn't say that you were a close friend of theirs. Gerald Wells and his wife Margaret were close to Nick and Joanne. Gerald was one of the other family physicians at the BFMC. Maybe Nick had called you instead of Gerald because you were close enough to him to be trusted but not so close as to prevent things from getting muddied in personal issues and allegiances. Probably it was because he knew that you already knew a lot about what had happened in his past, and the fewer who knew about that the better.

Nick had called at about 5:30 PM on Monday, July 3, about 10 days after his disappearance. You were in your office writing up charts on your computer at the end of the day. All the staff had gone home except for Jennifer Ling, one of the nurses. Jenny had answered the phone and put it through to your office. You were startled at first when Nick identified himself. He said he knew this must be a great surprise for you and asked you straight off not to call the police. He said he had not killed Amy Stephens but thought he might know who was behind it. He also said he had called his father, Alex, on the evening of June 30. That was the same day Alex had been in to see you and had told you all about the past events involving Nick and Amy. Only Alex, Cecilia, and Joanne knew he was alive and well. He said he needed your help but could not talk on the phone. He asked if you and he could meet somewhere private. You had been planning to go to Kingston on Wednesday and so you arranged to meet him in the Bracken Library.

As you drove now, you wondered if you had made the right decision. You wanted to believe he was telling the truth and from what you knew of him you found it difficult to believe he was a murderer. Still, people had been fooled in the past through naiveté. Perhaps you should have called the police. You would make up your mind after talking to him. Surely a public place like the medical library was safe. He wouldn't try anything there. Why would he have reason to hurt you anyway?

You had left Bedford at 12:30 PM, and by 2 PM you were sitting at a table in the basement floor of the library, as prearranged. This was the floor where all the periodicals were kept, and people were busy, looking for articles and photocopying. It was safe there, but you chose a table away from the bustle as he had requested. You had arranged to meet at 2:30 PM, so he wasn't there yet. You spent the 30 minutes looking for articles on diabetes and gonorrhea.

At 2:25 PM, Nick arrived. Dressed in jeans and a polo shirt, he was sporting a mustache that he had not had before. His hair was also a different color, jet black rather than the usual brown. You recognized him easily, but it was a good disguise for someone looking for a brown-haired man without a mustache. He sat down and thanked you for showing up as promised. You listened as he told his story.

The trip to Labrador had been a bit strained. Nick had originally planned to ask one of his law partners to go with him, but Nancy had practically begged him to invite Pierre instead. She really wanted Pierre and Nick to become friends. Things had always been a bit cool between them. Nick didn't really believe Pierre loved Nancy and felt the marriage was one forced by circumstances, with Nancy getting pregnant. He also had heard some vague rumors of infidelity on Pierre's part but had no proof of that. He just didn't like Pierre for reasons he couldn't always articulate or logically explain. Cecilia, who was Nick's and Nancy's mother, thought that Nick and Pierre were great friends, but she just didn't see beneath the veneer of civility that they displayed toward each other during family gatherings. Despite this, the trip had been a great experience and worth doing again some time.

Nick didn't know for certain why Pierre had wanted to drive to Toronto in separate cars when they left for Labrador, but apparently he had some business to attend to as soon as they arrived back. Nick had called Joanne from Goose Bay to let her know they were out of the bush safely. Their plane arrived back in Toronto at about 6 PM. They collected their gear from the baggage carousel and went to their individual cars. Pierre had been driving out of the parking garage just as Nick was about to open the trunk of his car. What he found when he opened the trunk was different in one significant way compared with what his father and later the police had found in the trunk.

There was an envelope sitting on the body bag. It had nothing written on the outside, but inside a typewritten letter read: "I know all about your little secret. You won't have to worry about her blackmailing you anymore, will you? But now you have me to worry about. So now we work by my plan. Meet me at the corner of Dundas and Yonge at 8 PM. Don't be stupid and go to the police. The body is in your car, and I'll see to it they find out about your secret, which they'll see as a motive for the murder. So leave the car where it is, and take a taxi to Dundas and Yonge. If we strike a new deal, I'll look after the body for you. And $25,000 won't be enough now."

I wasn't certain what to do at first. Should I call the police anyway? Should I just drive out of the parking garage and get rid of the body somewhere myself? It certainly was Amy Stephens' body in my trunk. I recognized her even with the swollen blue face and the strangulation marks around her neck. I tried to sort it out in my mind. From the letter, it seemed that someone had found out about Amy's blackmail of me and my payout of $25,000. They had then killed Amy and set it up to look like I may have done it by stuffing the body in my trunk. There would be no good proof that I had committed the murder, however, and no obvious motive unless the police found out about my previous relationship with Amy and the blackmail episode.

I decided to do as the writer of the letter had said. I took a taxi to Dundas and Yonge. The problem was the letter gave me no hint who I was looking for, what he was wearing, or what he would say to identify himself. It was as if the person assumed I would know all these things. I didn't! I walked around the intersection until 10 PM seeing no one I recognized. I approached a few people with the pretense of asking directions and tried to drop hints about the letter or say I was waiting to meet someone, but no one gave any hint of recognition. By 10 PM, I was tired and decided to check into a hotel for the night. Despite the events of the evening, I slept well. The trip to Labrador had been exhausting.

The next morning I didn't wake up until 11 AM. After a quick breakfast, I took a taxi to the airport. As I approached the parking level where my car had been I saw police around and my father speaking with one of them. I went on up to the next level and then back down to ground level and took a taxi back to the hotel.

Since then, I have stayed out of sight. I made my way to Kingston, started growing a mustache, and dyed my hair. I spent my time watching the papers. I knew the body had been identified as Amy Stephens and that she had been strangled. I knew I was a suspect and that the police were looking for me. I have a thousand questions. Who had found out about the blackmail episode, and how? How did they get into my car without seeming to break in? It was as if they had keys. If they had keys, how did they get them? Why didn't the security cameras in the garage see anyone stuffing a full-sized body into the trunk of a car. The car didn't seem to have left the parking garage during my 2 weeks away because the ticket stamped with June 9 was still on the dash. I had checked it that evening when I arrived back from Labrador, and it had been reported in the papers. If the person who had done it wanted to blackmail me, as it seemed from the letter, then why didn't they show up at the rendezvous place? Why hadn't they given me some indication of who or what I was looking for? It was a mystery within a mystery.

Nick finally got to the part you were wondering about as much as all the rest. Why had he contacted you?

Nick said he wanted to stop running and turn himself in to the police. But before he did that, he wanted to know that there was a possible alternate explanation that the police could pursue or already were pursuing. Providing them with a motive when he was already a suspect was asking for a guilty verdict. But if there was some other possible explanation to this, then he would take the chance. He was tired of being a fugitive, and he knew it was hurting his family. This is where you came in. He asked if you would be the channel through which he got messages to his family because he couldn't risk contacting them anymore with the police watching. He also asked you to try to find out two things for him. From Mrs. Stephens, Amy's mother, who lived in Bedford, he needed to know if there was anyone Amy had been dating recently who might have had a motive to kill her. He also needed to know from Sergeant FitzPatrick, the police officer in charge of the Bedford part of the investigation, whether there were other suspects and just how much the police knew. Both of these people were your patients, and he knew they were coming in to see you the next day. He didn't say how he knew, but you realized someone working in the clinic must have let him know. Someone else at the clinic was helping Nick as well!

You had great reservations about all of this. He was asking you to assist a murder suspect who was being sought by the police. This didn't sound like a good idea on the surface of it! He did say he would turn himself in once he had more information and could see a reasonable defense case building for himself. Maybe he was thinking like a lawyer, but running seemed to only make him look guilty. Maybe you trusted the law enforcement and legal systems more than he did. Perhaps he was a better judge of that. Whatever your final reasoning, and you weren't certain it was anything but a gut feeling that Nick was innocent and telling the truth, you agreed to try to find out the information he wanted. He didn't make you promise not to turn him in. You guessed he just had to trust you on that one. The plan was that he would call you again in 2 days, on Friday, at 5:30 PM.

This all took about an hour. Nick left and you spent a few hours searching the literature and copying articles. But your mind wasn't on the task. Your head was still spinning on the way home to Bedford. You didn't go home but crashed at Jonathon Simple's house for a few hours. Jon was one of the other physicians who worked in the clinic with you. You couldn't tell him anything of what had happened in Kingston, but you had a couple of beers together, chatted about some interesting cases, and then you went home. You smiled as you left remembering that Jon always said that all he wanted to be was a "simple family doctor." You and Jon were the single docs in your group. The married physicians and your other friends always were trying to find partners for you, but neither of you were interested. Work took up most of your time.

ACT II

Beatrice's Grief
(Hypothyroidism)

Beatrice Stephens, Amy's mother, arrived at your office the day after your meeting with Nick. Beatrice had moved back to Bedford 2 years ago after her husband died. The family had lived in Bedford until Amy was 14 years old. They were never very well off and had left Kingston when Tom, Beatrice's husband, found a better job in Toronto.

Beatrice was already on thyroid replacement hormone when you first saw her 2 years ago. She was one of those people who seemed to need to be maintained at a slightly hyperthyroid level to feel well. The thyroid-stimulating hormone (TSH) level she had measured 2 days ago was 0.3 mU/L (normal range 0.25–5.0 mU/L) with a free thyroxine (FT_4) level of 0.25 (normal range 9–25 pmol/L). Normally, you would recommend that she cut back from her thyroxine dose of 1.5 mg to about 1.25 mg in this situation, but you had been down that road before. Each time you cut back her dose, she started complaining of extreme fatigue. At the higher level of FT_4, her pulse runs around 80–85 beats/min, and her blood pressure is 145/90 mm Hg. It didn't change appreciably when you had lowered her thyroid replacement dose in the past. You have always wondered if she was just someone who needed a level outside the usual normal range to be euthyroid "for her." She had a fairly strong family history of coronary heart disease, however, and you also wondered if the elevated FT_4 could lead to trouble if it was causing a positive chronotropic effect on the heart.

Beatrice wasn't too concerned about her thyroid or much else about herself today. Amy, who had been her only child, had been buried in Toronto about a week ago. Beatrice now felt alone in the world. You talked with her a while. She wanted to go over the whole thing. She had been visiting Amy for a few days and was there on the day she died. Amy had received a call in the morning of the day she died. She told her mother she had to go visit someone for a short while in the afternoon. At about 1 pm, a man showed up in a dark red BMW; Amy said goodbye and that she would be back in an hour. Looking out through the window, Beatrice saw the driver get out of the car as Amy approached. He chatted with Amy for a minute standing by the car, then Amy and the man got in the car and they drove off. There was also another man in the car, but Beatrice didn't really see his face. She never saw Amy alive again.

She thought she could identify the man if she saw him again. She had sat with a police artist, and a picture was sketched, but Beatrice didn't think it had really captured his looks. She said she found it difficult describing people.

Beatrice said Amy had been seeing a man from Bedford, but that it had broken off 4 months earlier. Amy hadn't seemed saddened by it and already had dated several other men. She didn't have a problem finding men, it seemed. This bothered Beatrice. She thought Amy had perhaps not been as discerning of men as she should be and was often taken advantage of. Beatrice tried to talk to her about this, but Amy would just laugh and tell her she was being careful and things were fine. Beatrice worried she would become pregnant again and have an abortion like she did 10 years ago. She didn't know who the father had been at that time and mentioned nothing about any money coming to Amy. She knew the father had been from Bedford, and she wondered if the man from Bedford she had been dating up until 4 months ago was the same man.

Amy had never married. She had been 22 years old when she had the abortion and 32 when she died. Beatrice had no grandchildren and wishes now she had agreed to care for the baby and perhaps Amy wouldn't have had an abortion. Perhaps things would have been different, and she wouldn't be dead now. All of these things were going through Beatrice's mind. The "what ifs." What if she had done something differently? What if she had discouraged Amy from leaving in that car on that last day? It was the usual and understandable grief and subtle self-blaming that many grieving people experience. You assured her that there was nothing she could have done that likely would have changed things. You encouraged her to think of the good times and the beautiful things in Amy's life and their life together as a family.

You wondered if Beatrice had told Sergeant FitzPatrick or the Toronto police about the previous abortion and about the father being from Bedford?

Some questions arising from this clinical encounter

19 In a 61-year-old woman on thyroid replacement therapy and a family history of coronary heart disease but no symptoms herself, does maintaining her FT_4 at a level slightly above the usual normal range put her at risk of adverse cardiovascular outcomes?

20 Are there factors to predict whether a grief reaction after a loss will become prolonged and pathologic?

Reflection Exercise:

What are your thoughts regarding these questions? Consider them in the context of your own practice. Consider what you might do before you read the evidence.

Preamble

We found two studies that addressed this question.

Citation: Peters A, Ehlers M, Blank B, et al. Excess triiodothyronine as a risk factor for coronary events. Arch Intern Med 2000; 160:1993–1998.[81]

Study design: Cross-sectional study and prospective cohort substudy.

Study population: All (1049) patients ≥40 years old presenting to the emergency department at the Medical University of Lubeck from January 1 to April 30, 1995, were included in the cross-sectional study. A subpopulation (181) of this group who had a diagnosis of angina or acute myocardial infarction were followed subsequently for 3 years.

Data collected: Free triiodothyronine (T_3), free T_4, and TSH were collected on all patients as they arrived in the emergency department. Angina pectoris and acute myocardial infarction were diagnosed based on symptoms, electrocardiogram classification, cardiac enzymes, and patient history related to coronary heart disease. Of the 185 patients with angina or acute myocardial infarction, 181 were followed for 3 years.

Follow-up: The 3-year cohort outcomes were occurrence of acute myocardial infarction in patients who had angina on admission and occurrence of death or recurrent acute myocardial infarction in patients who had acute myocardial infarction on admission.

The Evidence: Effect of Elevated Free Triiodothyronine

Outcome	EER (Outcome in Those with Elevated FT$_3$)	CER (Outcome in Those with Normal FT$_3$)	Relative Risk	ARI	NNEh
Angina or AMI at time of admission	17 of 60 (0.28)	168 of 989 (0.17)	1.67 (1.6–1.73)	11%	9
AMI or death during 3-year cohort follow-up	5 of 16 (0.31)	17 of 142 (0.12)	2.9 (2.6–3.3)	19%	5

EER, experimental event rate; FT3, free triiodothyronine; CER, control event rate; ARI, absolute risk increase; NNEh, number needed to be exposed to harm 1 person; AMI, acute myocardial infarction.

The Evidence: Effect of Elevated Free Thyrokine

Outcome	EER (Outcome in Those with Elevated FT₄)	CER (Outcome in Those with Normal FT₄)	Relative Risk	ARR	NNEb
Angina or AMI at time of admission	17 of 99 (0.172)	168 of 950 (0.177)	0.97 (0.96–0.98)	0.5%	200
AMI or death during 3-year cohort follow-up	2 of 17 (0.118)	20 of 164 (0.122)	0.96 (0.95–0.99)	0.4%	250

EER, experimental event rate; CER, control event rate; ARR, absolute risk reduction; NNEb, number needed to be exposed to benefit 1 person; FT_4, free thyroxine; AMI, acute myocardial infarction.

The Evidence: Effect of Suppressed Thyroid-Stimulating Hormone

Outcome	EER (Outcome in Those with Suppressed TSH)	CER (Outcome in Those without Suppressed TSH)	Relative Risk	ARR	NNEb
Angina or AMI at time of admission	14 of 108 (0.13)	171 of 941 (0.18)	0.71 (0.69–0.74)	5%	20
AMI or death during 3-year cohort follow-up	5 of 35 (0.2)	17 of 156 (0.11)	1.8 (1.7–2.0)	−9%	−11

EER, experimental event rate; TSH, thyroid-stimulating hormone; CER, control event rate, ARR, absolute risk reduction; NNEb, number needed to be exposed to benefit 1 person; AMI, acute myocardial infarction.

Interpretation: This study reveals a mixed picture. Elevated free T_3, essentially T_3 thyrotoxicosis, seems to be a significant risk factor for ischemic heart disease. Elevated free T_4 is not associated with increased risk of ischemic heart disease, however, and may have a slight beneficial effect. Suppressed TSH seems to have an adverse effect when it is acutely suppressed but not over the longer term.

Bottom line: Elevated free T_3 is a risk factor for ischemic cardiac events. Whether elevated T_4 or suppressed TSH is also a risk factor is questionable.

Citation: Leese GP, Jung RT, Guthrie C, et al. Morbidity in patients on L-thyroxine: A comparison of those with a normal TSH to those with suppressed TSH. Clin Endocrinol 1992; 37:500–503.[59]

Study design: Cross-sectional study of disease incidence by TSH level.

Study population: A total of 1180 patients from Tayside, Scotland, with hypothyroidism who were on thyroid hormone replacement.

Data collection: All 1180 patients were seen during a 1-year period and had thyroid function tests. Morbidity data from the Tayside Thyroid Registry were used to assess the outcomes in patients with normal TSH and suppressed TSH.

Outcomes considered: Ischemic heart disease, overall fractures, fractures of the neck of the femur, and breast carcinoma.

The evidence: Of the 1180 patients, 58.5% (691) had suppressed TSH, and 38% (448) had normal TSH. These patients (1144) comprised the overall sample for the comparisons made in the study. Patients with suppressed TSH had overall higher serum T_4 levels, as would be expected.

The authors do not provide sufficient information to recalculate and confirm their results. We can only present their data as they have done and from that determine absolute risk reduction and number needed to be exposed. The relative risk and 95% confidence interval cannot be determined. We are assuming the authors are correct in their estimation of statistical significance. They state that low TSH did not affect the incidence of any of the outcomes considered (ischemic heart disease, fractures, and breast carcinoma).

The Evidence: Effect of Suppressed Thyroid-Stimulating Hormone on Incidence of Ischemic Heart Disease

Outcome	EER (Outcome in Those with Suppressed TSH)	CER (Outcome in Those with Normal TSH)	Relative Risk	ARR	NNEb
Ischemic heart disease (age ≤ 65 y)	2.8%	3.4%	Unable to calculate	NA	NA
Ischemic heart disease (age >65 y)	4.2%	4.2%	Unable to calculate	NA	NA

EER, experimental event rate; TSH, thyroid-stimulating hormone; CER, control event rate; ARR, absolute risk reduction; NNEb, number needed to be exposed to benefit 1 person; NA, not applicable as there is no significant difference.

Interpretation: This study does not find any association between presence of suppressed TSH in patients on thyroid hormone replacement therapy and the incidence of ischemic heart disease, fractures, or breast cancer.

Bottom line: Patients on hormone replacement therapy with suppressed TSH are not at significantly higher risk for ischemic heart disease.

Overall summary: It probably is safe to maintain a slightly elevated T_4 and suppressed TSH in patients on thyroid replacement therapy who feel better at a higher replacement level of T_4. It might be wise, however, to measure the free T_3 level because an elevated free T_3 level may be associated with adverse outcomes.

What did Dr. Sharpe do?

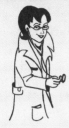

Mrs. Stephens does not have heart disease, although there is a family history. Mrs. Stephens' blood pressure and pulse are not elevated with the increased T_4 levels. Given the information in these studies, Dr. Sharpe decided to keep Mrs. Stephens on 1.5 mg of T_4, to monitor her clinically for signs of overstimulation, and to check her free T_3 level.

Reflection Exercise: How does this evidence apply to your practice? Would you apply this evidence to the management of appropriate patients in your practice? How will your practice change?

Answer to Question 20

Preamble

We were unable to find a study that takes an evidence-based approach to answering this question. We were looking for a study that prospectively (or retrospectively) assessed various demographic and relationship factors before the death and correlated these with occurrence or degree of pathologic grief. The closest we found were three studies that addressed the issue from different viewpoints.

Citation: Shanfield SB, Benjamin H, Swain BJ. Parents' reactions to the death of an adult child from cancer. Am J Psychiatry 1984; 141:1092–1094.[93]

Study design: Survey.

Study population: The charts of 215 patients <60 years old who had died at a hospice were reviewed to 4 years after death. Of these, 30 had surviving parents who could be contacted. These parents were sent questionnaires. A total of 24 parents of 18 deceased children responded. The average age of the parents at time of death of the adult child was 63 years. The average age of the adult child at the time of death was 39 years. All died of cancer.

Data collection: The questionnaire sought information about the parent and his or her relationship with the adult child during the illness. In addition, the Brief Symptom Inventory was asked to be completed and a validated self-report inventory that measures psychiatric symptoms.

Results: Parents who felt close to their children had a more intense grief reaction and less guilt. They also reported less unfinished business with the children at the time of death. A relationship between parent and child characterized by negative feelings increased psychiatric symptoms during the bereavement period.

Interpretation: The relationship between parent and child is an important factor in the bereavement process of parents who lose adult children.

Bottom line: Parents who have had a positive relationship with their child will have fewer psychiatric symptoms during the bereavement period after that child's death.

Citation: Horowitz MJ, Siegel B, Holen A, et al. Diagnostic criteria for complicated grief disorder. Am J Psychiatry 1997; 154:905–910.[46]

Note: The authors conducted the process outlined in this article to develop diagnostic criteria for the classification of a separate disorder in DSM-V called *Complicated Grief Disorder.* This disorder is not in DSM-IV. The condition is subsumed under posttraumatic distress syndrome.

Study design: Clinical interview.

Study population: Ninety subjects, 6 months after their loss of a long-term domestic partner, were evaluated. There were 29 men and 61 women.

Data collection: Numerous clinical symptoms were evaluated under the categories of avoidance (e.g., low interest in important activities), intrusion (e.g., unbidden memories), and failure to adapt (e.g., feeling of life being on hold). These symptoms were assessed at 6 months and 14 months after the death of the loved one.

Results: Proposed diagnostic criteria for complicated grief disorder

A. Event criterion/prolonged response criterion. Bereavement (loss of a spouse, other relative, or intimate partner) at least 14 months ago (12 months is avoided because of possible intense turbulence from an anniversary reaction).
B. Signs and symptoms criteria. In the last month, any three of the following seven symptoms with a severity that interferes with daily functioning.
   Intrusive symptoms:
   1. Unbidden memories or intrusive fantasies related to the lost relationship.
   2. Strong spells or pangs of severe emotion related to the lost relationship.
   3. Distressingly strong yearnings or wishes that the deceased were there.
   Signs of avoidance and failure to adapt:
   4. Feelings of being too much alone or personally empty.
   5. Excessively staying away from people, places, or activities that remind the subject of the deceased.
   6. Unusual levels of sleep interference.
   7. Loss of interest in work, social, caretaking, or recreational activities to a maladaptive degree.

Interpretation: Explicit clinical criteria for the diagnosis of pathologic grief or Complicated Grief Disorder have been developed.

Citation: Sheldon F. ABC of palliative care: Bereavement. BMJ 1998; 216:456–458.[94]

Note: This is an opinion article based on experience with bereaved patients. It does address most directly, however, the clinical question we are asking. Risk factors for a poor outcome of bereavement are listed.

Risk factors for poor outcome of bereavement

Predisposing factors
- Ambivalent or dependent relationship
- Multiple prior bereavements
- Previous mental illness, especially depression
- Low self-esteem of bereaved person

Around time of death
- Sudden and unexpected death
- Untimely death of young person
- Preparation for the death
- Stigmatized deaths—such as AIDS, suicide
- Culpable deaths
- Sex of bereaved person—elderly male widower
- Caring for the deceased person for >6 months
- Inability to carry out valued religious rituals

After the death
- Level of perceived social support
- Lack of opportunities for new interests
- Stress from other life crises

Interpretation: A useful list is provided of considerations when trying to determine a person's risk of a pathologic grief reaction. The degree to which this list is accurate is unknown, however, because no evidence is quoted in the development of the list.

Summary of results of the three articles: The relationship between the bereaved parent and the dead child, especially around the time before the death, seems to be important in predicting whether the bereavement process will be "normal." Specific criteria are available to diagnose Complicated Grief Disorder. Professionals who deal with bereaved people are able to cite factors that may predict a poor outcome and result in Complicated Grief Disorder.

What did Dr. Sharpe do?

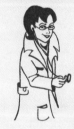

Dr. Sharpe decided she should ask Mrs. Stephens to come back in for a visit to talk things over. She would assess the sort of relationship Mrs. Stephens and Amy had as mother and daughter, determine if there was any "unfinished business," let Mrs. Stephens talk about things, and perhaps refer her to a bereavement support group if one existed in Bedford. Dr. Sharpe also would follow Mrs. Stephens closely over the next year or so to watch for the symptoms of Complicated Grief Disorder.

Reflection Exercise: How does this evidence apply to your practice? Would you apply this evidence to the management of appropriate patients in your practice? How will your practice change?

Aunt Joan's Rumor
(Congestive Heart Failure)

Joan Walters is 75 years old and the oldest sister of Matt Walters, Joanne Walters-Sampson's father. Joan was a bit of a busybody and liked to find out everybody else's business, one of the biggest gossips in town. If you wanted something to "get around," just let it slip to "Aunt Joan." Everybody seemed to call her Aunt Joan, whether she was their aunt or not.

Joan had become your patient just 3 years ago, after her previous physician died. For a while you thought she was going to outlive you as well, but then she had a mild heart attack. Combined with 20 years of poorly controlled hypertension, the myocardial infarction had led to subsequent development of congestive heart failure (CHF). She was on digoxin, 0.125 mg daily, and furosemide, 20 mg daily. A colleague had given a presentation on CHF a few weeks ago and had said that all patients with CHF should be on an angiotensin-converting enzyme (ACE) inhibitor. You wondered if it applied in this case, in which the patient seemed perfectly controlled on digoxin and furosemide.

Today Aunt Joan's blood pressure was 150/90 mm Hg, and her pulse was 75 beats/min. Her chest was clear, and there was just a trace of pedal edema, probably more due to venous stasis then CHF. She admitted to getting short of breath if she hurried or went upstairs, and she liked to sleep with her head high, although she didn't wake up at night short of breath.

Despite her reputation for gossiping (or maybe because of it!), you like Aunt Joan and would like her to be around for a while. You wonder if there are factors that predict outcome in CHF and whether you can alter these factors to improve outcomes.

Aunt Joan decides she wants to tell you all about the murder mystery that is on the go in Bedford, as if you haven't heard! You normally would try politely to avoid having to listen and find a way to get on to your next patient, but today you decide to listen. She tells you all about the mysterious circumstances of the body in Nick's car and his disappearance. She tells you that Amy Stephens used to live in Bedford years ago and that

> she was a "wild one" even as a young teenager. There were stories of her running around with older men at all hours of the night. Her parents couldn't control her at all. They left Bedford because of some sort of scandal with her mother who has since come back to Bedford, you know! Joanne's Nick was mixed up with her about 10 years ago. Apparently got her pregnant, but she had an abortion. Joanne doesn't know anything about this, so Nick thinks, but everybody knows really, probably Joanne too. Robert Stenson sees to that. Him and Stefan Richard tell stories about what goes on in those

families you know. I don't know about those two, running off to Toronto together like that. People say they are homosexual you know. But anyway it's not only Nick who has had a run-in with Amy Stephens. I hear Pierre Savoy was having an affair with her, behind Nancy's back. I wonder if he isn't involved in this whole mess somehow. I never liked that Pierre Savoy. He's been up to no good since he was a boy. I remember the time when he was just a teenager and he beat up one of the boys working in his father's store. Blamed the poor boy for stealing when all he was doing was running an errand for Mr. Savoy himself. It's not beyond Pierre Savoy to try to get Nick in trouble even if he is married to his sister. Especially after that court case that Nick won for that poor man against the Savoy Supermarket. They aren't very good to the people working for them you know.

Your head was still spinning as she left. But you were glad you had listened. You had not heard about this affair between Amy and Pierre before. Maybe Pierre was the man from Bedford that Beatrice had talked about. If so, the relationship had broken off 4 months ago according to Beatrice. If that was so, there was the making of a case against Pierre Savoy with a motive of rejected love. A bit thin! Especially with the body showing up in Nick's car and a letter written to Nick placed in the trunk. Perhaps Pierre had the body planted there to get revenge on Nick for that lost court case you had heard about previously, which did lose the Savoys about $100,000—maybe not a lot of money in their terms, but enough just the same. You wondered why you were suspecting Pierre. There was nothing but rumors to implicate him. Maybe that lie he told about his injury still bothered you a bit. You wondered how his leg was.

You laughed as you thought of Aunt Joan's reference to Robert Stensen and Stefan Richard; Stensen was the butler and driver for the Sampsons, and Richard was the butler and driver for the Savoys. It was true what she said about them being lovers and spending their free time together in Toronto, but for her to be accusing them of gossiping seemed laughable!

Some questions arising from this clinical encounter

21 In a 75-year-old woman with CHF well controlled on digoxin and furosemide, would adding an ACE inhibitor to her medication regimen provide any benefit?

22 Which factors predict 5-year outcome in elderly people with CHF?

_____

Reflection Exercise

What are your thoughts regarding these questions? Consider them in the context of your own practice. Consider what you might do before you read the evidence.

Citation: Flather MD, Yusuf S, Kober L, et al. Long-term ACE-inhibitor therapy in patients with heart failure or left-ventricular dysfunction: A systematic review of data from individual patients. Lancet 2000; 355:1575–1581.[26]

Study design: Systematic review with pooling of individual patient data.

Data sources: Medline, hand searching of reference lists.

Number of studies: 3

Number of patients: 5966

Time frame: 1990s

Article selection criteria: Randomized controlled trials of >1000 patients that compared ACE inhibitors with controls after myocardial infarction for at least 12 months and that did an intention-to-treat analysis.

Data extraction: The datasets of the three trials were obtained and combined and reanalyzed as a single dataset.

Article appraisal process: NA.

Statistical heterogeneity tests? NA.

Publication bias testing? NA

Other study details: The three trials were SAVE (Survival and Ventricular Enlargement), AIRE (Acute Infarction Ramipril Efficacy), and TRACE (Trandolapril in Patients with Reduced Left Ventricular Function After Acute Myocardial Infarction). The intent was to compare the results of the pooled data from these trials with the data from the SOLVD (Studies of Left Ventricular Dysfunction) trials. The three trials consisted of 76% men and 24% women. Mean age was 63 years. Mean ejection fraction was 32%. Mean follow-up time was 31 months. Other drugs taken by the participants included aspirin in 75%, diuretics in 52%, and β-blockers in 25%.

The Evidence

Outcome	EER (ACE Inhibitor)	CER (Placebo)	Peto Odds Ratio	ARR	NNTb
Death	702 of 2995 (23.4%)	866 of 2971 (29.1%)	0.74 (0.66–0.83)	5.7%	18
Readmission for heart failure	355 of 2995 (11.9%)	460 of 2971 (15.5%)	0.73 (0.63–0.85)	3.6%	28
Reinfarction	324 of 2995 (10.8%)	391 of 2971 (13.2%)	0.80 (0.69–0.94)	2.4%	42

EER, experimental event rate; ACE, angiotensin-converting enzyme; CER, control even rate; ARR, absolute risk reduction; NNTb, number needed to treat to benefit 1 person.

Interpretation: The participants included patients on other drugs and subjects who were not on any medication. They were not all exactly like the case in question, in which the patient already was on furosemide and digoxin. The results are striking, however. Similar to the SOLVD studies, this review found that taking an ACE inhibitor after a myocardial infarction decreased the likelihood of subsequent admission for CHF and of reinfarction and death. The numbers needed to treat are not too large considering the seriousness of the outcomes. The most serious outcome, death, had the lowest number needed to treat.

Bottom line: In patients who have had a myocardial infarction, taking an ACE inhibitor decreases the likelihood of death, reinfarction, and admission for CHF for at least 3 years after myocardial infarction.

What did Dr. Sharpe do?

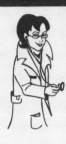

Dr. Sharpe added ramipril to Aunt Joan's medication regimen. She chose ramipril because it was the ACE inhibitor used in one of the three trials included in this review and because of the data from the HOPE trial, which further supported the usefulness of ramipril.

Reflection Exercise: How does this evidence apply to your practice? Would you apply this evidence to the management of appropriate patients in your practice? How will your practice change?

Answer to Question 22

Citation: Kalon KL, Anderson KM, Kannel WB, et al. Survival after onset of congestive heart failure in Framingham Heart Study subjects. Circulation 1993; 88:107–115.[52]

Study design: Longitudinal cohort study: the Framingham Study.

Patient population: The patients who were enrolled in the Framingham Study (N = 5209) in 1948 and their offspring (N = 5135), who were enrolled in 1972. Of these, 9405 were eligible for analysis.

Follow-up: The 9405 patients were followed a median length of 14.8 years. During this time, 652 patients developed CHF. These 652 patients constituted the follow-up cohort for this study.

Data collection: The original cohort enrolled in 1948 were assessed initially, then every 2 years. The offspring cohort was assessed initially, then after 8 and 12 years. At each examination, cardiovascular disease events were identified by medical history, physical examination, 12-lead electrocardiogram, and review of medical records.

The Evidence: Changing Age of First Diagnosis of Congestive Heart Failure Over the Decades

Decade	Mean Age of Diagnosis of CHF
1950s	57
1960s	66
1970s	72
1980s	76
Overall	70
Overall women	72
Overall men	68

The 652 patients with CHF were followed for a mean of 3.9 years (SD 5.4 years). There were 551 deaths, for an overall death rate of 84.5%.

The Evidence

Time after onset of CHF (y)	Survival Rate in Women (%)	Survival Rate in Men (%)
1	64	57
2	56	46
5	38	25
10	21	11

In men, CHF secondary to valvular heart disease carried a worse prognosis compared with CHF secondary to coronary heart disease (hazards ratio, 1.68; 95% confidence interval, 1.15–2.46). This was not the case in women. Survival in women was worse, however, if they had diabetes (hazards ratio, 1.7; 95% confidence interval, 1.21–2.38) or if they had left ventricular hypertrophy (hazards ratio, 1.63; 95% confidence interval, 1.08–2.45). There was no difference in the survival rate from CHF over the 40-year period of observation.

Finally, the study authors looked at the survival rates of people who survived the first 90 days after first diagnoses. In other words, if a patient survived the first 3 months after the diagnosis and was over the acute event of whatever triggered it, what were the survival rates? In these people, the median survival rate was 3.2 years in men and 4.4 years in women. The following table gives the rates at 1, 2, 5, and 10 years.

The Evidence: Survival Rates in Patients Still Alive 90 Days After Diagnosis of Congestive Heart Failure

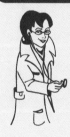

Time After Onset of CHF (y)	Survival Rate in Women (%)	Survival Rate in Men (%)
1	88	79
2	78	63
5	53	25
10	29	15

Interpretation: Better medical care, decreased smoking rates, lowering of cholesterol, and controlling blood pressure have made a difference in the time of onset of CHF, as the average age went from about 57 years old in the 1950s to 76 years old in the 1980s. When a person got CHF, however, their survival rate was no better in the 1980s than it was in the 1950s; 47–75% are dead within 5 years (depending on their sex and on whether or not they survive the early months after diagnosis). It is interesting to speculate whether these rates will have improved for the 1990s and the first decade of the twenty-first century with the use of ACE inhibitors, which have been shown to decrease the death rate from CHF.

Bottom line: The 5-year survival rate after diagnosis of CHF is 38% for women and 25% for men. If they survive the first 90 days after diagnosis, the subsequent survival rate is better—53% for women and 35% for men.

What did Dr. Sharpe do?

Dr. Sharpe found these results interesting. She had not realized it was quite that bad. She decided that prevention was the key and that she should make an effort to prevent her patients from getting CHF in the first place. She wondered if the results would be better now that ACE inhibitors have been shown to decrease death rates. She was glad she decided to start Aunt Joan on ramipril.

Reflection Exercise: How does this evidence apply to your practice? Would you apply this evidence to the management of appropriate patients in your practice? How will your practice change?

Fitz
(Ischemic Heart Disease)

Sergeant Sean FitzPatrick, or Fitz as everyone called him, was well known and liked in Bedford. He was with the Ontario Provincial Police, who provided policing services for Bedford. Fitz wasn't running the Amy Stephens investigation; that was being done out of Toronto, but he was assigned to the Bedford end of the case.

Fitz had had a triple coronary artery bypass graft operation 2 years ago. He came from a family with a strong history of ischemic heart disease. His father and grandfather had died in their 50s of heart attacks. His older brother was severely incapacitated at age 58 years, having had two myocardial infarctions and a bypass operation. He was now in severe heart failure and was being considered for a heart transplant.

Fitz worried about this a lot. He wanted to do everything he could to prevent ending up like his brother. He had quit smoking and drinking. He was doing well on a diet and was walking 5 km every day. He was doing so well you felt obliged to do everything you could. He had two other risk factors, hypertension and hyperlipidemia.

Today his blood pressure was 150/92 mm Hg. That seemed reasonably good, but you wondered what his ideal blood pressure should be. How far should you push his blood pressure down with medication? He was on hydrochlorothiazide, 25 mg daily, and atenolol, 25 mg daily.

You had the results of his most recent fasting lipid profile. His total cholesterol is 5.8 mmol/L, low-density lipoprotein (LDL) is 3.0 mmol/L, and high-density lipoprotein (HDL) is 1.0 mmol/L; his total cholesterol-to-HDL ratio is 5.8. His triglycerides are at 2.8 mmol/L. He is on simvastatin, 10 mg daily. You know these numbers could be better, but again how far should you go; what should the goal of treatment be?

You ask Fitz how the Amy Stephens investigation is going, explaining your interest was because of the effect the whole situation was having on the Sampson family, many of whom were your patients. Fitz says they are still looking for Nick Sampson. Their latest information is that he is in Kingston, but they haven't located him yet. He says that Nick's running makes him look like a guilty man—if he is running, that is. There is always the possibility that he is dead. They know that Amy died of strangulation at about 2 PM the day Nick and Pierre arrived back from Labrador. Since their plane didn't get in until 6 PM, it means neither of them could have done it themselves. He says, however, that with families like the Sampsons and Savoys, you always can get someone else to do the dirty work.

Nick's fingerprints were all over the garbage bag that contained Amy's body, but that's probably because he opened it to look in. Did he know who it would be before he opened that bag? If he did, it probably was because he had arranged the murder. If not, it probably was a surprise to him. In either case, why did he just take off and leave the car there? The best guess the police had was that he had arranged the murder but not that the body be stored in his car. They thought that the people who he contracted to do the murder had decided to turn the tables on him somehow by sticking him with the body. They think that he left the car where it was, so as not to run the risk of getting caught with the body, and went after the people who did it. His credit card was used in Kingston, which is what makes the police think he is there or at least heading east. It is also possible that someone killed him and has his credit card.

Fitz also mentioned that they had reason to believe he had known Amy Stephens in the past. She had become pregnant by him and had an abortion. He mentioned nothing about the blackmail, so you suspect he doesn't know about it. Fitz says, however, that this provides a link between Nick and Amy and a possible motive—although why he would have her killed 10 years later when it was all over and done makes no sense.

You thanked Fitz for chatting with you about it. He would be returning in a month.

Some questions arising from this clinical encounter

23 In a 53-year-old man with coronary artery disease (had a myocardial infarction 2 years ago) and with a strong family history of death from myocardial infarction in men in their 50s, what should be the target blood pressure for treatment of hypertension?

24 In a 53-year-old man with coronary artery disease (had a myocardial infarction 2 years ago) and with a strong family history of death from myocardial infarction in men in their 50s, what should be the target levels for treatment of hyperlipidemia?

Reflection Exercise:

What are your thoughts regarding these questions? Consider them in the context of your own practice. Consider what you might do before you read the evidence.

> Citation: Feldman RD, Campbell N, Larochelle P, et al. 1999 Canadian recommendations for the management of hypertension. Can Med Assoc J 1999; 161(12 Suppl):S1–S17. Also available at http://www.cma.ca/cmaj/vol-161/issue-12/hypertension/hyper-e.htm.[25]

Guideline objective: To provide updated, evidenced-based recommendations for health care professionals on the management of hypertension in adults.

Outcomes considered: Changes in blood pressure and in morbidity and mortality rates.

Data sources: Medline, scanning of reference lists, polling of experts, and the personal files of authors. All relevant articles were reviewed, classified according to design and graded to levels of evidence.

Recommendations pertinent to this question:
1. The diastolic blood pressure treatment goal is a pressure of <90 mm Hg. For systolic blood pressure, the goal is a pressure level of <140 mm Hg.
2. Hypertension in people with diabetes should be treated to obtain target blood pressure <130/80 mm Hg.

Interpretation: A target blood pressure of <140/90 mm Hg is recommended. This is based primarily on the results of the HOT trial (see later)

Bottom line: Blood pressure should be controlled to a level <140/90 mm Hg.

> Citation: Hansson L, Zanchetti A, Caruthers G, et al. Effects of intensive blood-pressure lowering and low-dose aspirin in patients with hypertension: Principal results of the Hypertension Optimal Treatment (HOT) randomized trial. Lancet 1998; 351:1755–1762.[38]

Study design: Randomized controlled trial, blinded, multicentered, with intention-to-treat analysis.

Sample size: 18,790

Study population: Patients from 26 countries in Europe, North and South America, and Asia were recruited between October 1992 until April 1994. The last day of follow-up was August 31, 1997. Average follow-up time was 3.8 years. Patients were aged 50–80 years with mean age of 61.5 years. All patients had hypertension with diastolic blood pressure 110–115 mm Hg (mean 105 mm Hg).

Randomization groups: First, patients were randomly assigned to one of three diastolic blood pressure target groups: ≤90 mm Hg, ≤85 mm Hg, ≤80 mm Hg with sample sizes of 6264, 6264, and 6262. Patients in each group were randomized in a double-blind manner to either low-dose aspirin (75 mg) or placebo. Of patients, 9399 received aspirin and 9391 received placebo.

Outcomes: The principal aims of the study were (1) to assess the association between major cardiovascular events and the target blood pressures (major cardiovascular events were nonfatal myocardial infarction, nonfatal stroke, and cardiovascular death), (2) to assess the association between major cardiovascular events and the diastolic blood pressures achieved during treatment, and (3) to determine whether the addition of low-dose aspirin to antihypertensive treatment reduces the rate of major cardiovascular events.

Other study details: Felodipine, 5 mg once daily, was given to all patients. Additional therapy and dose increments was given in four further steps to reach the randomized target blood pressure. Angiotensin-converting enzyme inhibitors or β-blockers were added at step 2, and dosage titrations were used at steps 3 and 4.

The Evidence: Target Group Differences in Cardiovascular Events

Outcome (Comparison)	EER (85 mm Hg Target)	CER (90 mm Hg Target)	Relative Risk	ARR	NNTb
All cardiovascular events (85 mm Hg vs 90 mm Hg)	234 of 6264 (3.7%)	232 of 6264 (3.7%)	0 (0.82–1.18)	NA	NA

	EER (80 mm Hg Target)	CER (90 mm Hg Target)	Relative Risk	ARR	NNTb
All cardiovascular events (80 mm Hg vs 90 mm Hg)	217 of 6262 (3.5%)	232 of 6264 (3.7%)	0.95 (0.77–1.0)	NA	NA

	EER (80 mm Hg Target)	CER (85 mm Hg Target)	Relative Risk	ARR	NNTb
All cardiovascular events (80 mm Hg vs 85 mm Hg)	217 of 6262 (3.5%)	234 of 6264 (3.7%)	0.95 (0.77–1.0)	NA	NA

EER, experimental event rate; CER, control event rate; ARR, absolute risk reduction; NNTb, number needed to treat to benefit 1 person; NA, not applicable as there is no significant difference.

The previous table shows that there was no difference in overall outcomes among the three target blood pressure groups. The same was true when the outcomes of myocardial infarction, stroke, and death were looked at individually.

The following table looks at outcomes in patients with diabetes in the three target blood pressure groups.

The Evidence: Target Group Differences in Cardiovascular Events in Diabetic Patients

Outcome (Comparison)	EER (85 mm Hg Target)	CER (90 mm Hg Target)	Relative Risk	ARR	NNTb
All cardiovascular events in diabetic patients (85 mm Hg vs 90 mm Hg)	34 of 501 (6.8%)	45 of 501 (9.0%)	0.76 (0.38–1.13)	NA	NA

Outcome (Comparison)	EER (80 mm Hg Target)	CER (90 mm Hg Target)	Relative Risk	ARR	NNTb
All cardiovascular events (80 mm Hg vs 90 mm Hg)	22 of 499 (4.4%)	45 of 501 (9.0%)	0.49 (0.15–0.83)	4.6%	22

Outcome (Comparison)	EER (80 mm Hg Target)	CER (85 mm Hg Target)	Relative Risk	ARR	NNTb
All cardiovascular events (80 mm Hg vs 85 mm Hg)	22 of 499 (4.4%)	34 of 501 (6.8)	0.65 (0.23–1.07)	NA	NA

EER, experimental event rate; CER, control event rate; ARR, absolute risk reduction; NNTb, number needed to treat to benefit 1 person; NA, not applicable as there is no significant difference.

The previous table shows a significant difference between the 90-mm Hg target group and the 80-mm Hg target group with fewer cardiovascular events in the 80-mm Hg target group. When the cardiovascular events were looked at individually, this effect was due mainly to a decreased cardiovascular death rate. The decreases in myocardial infarction and stroke did not reach statistical significance, although there was a trend in that direction.

The Evidence

Outcome	EER (Low-Dose Aspirin)	CER (Placebo)	Relative Risk	ARR	NNTb
All major cardiovascular events	315 of 9399 (3.4%)	368 of 9391 (3.9%)	0.85 (0.73–0.99)	0.5%	200
All myocardial infarction	82 of 9399 (0.9%)	127 of 9391 (1.4%)	0.64 (0.49–0.85)	0.5%	200
All stroke	146 of 9399	148 of 9391	0.98 (0.78–1.24)	NA	NA
Cardiovascular mortality	133 of 9399	140 of 9391	0.95 (0.75–1.20)	NA	NA

EER, experimental event rate; CER, control event rate; ARR, absolute risk reduction; NNTb, number related to treat to benefit 1 person; NA, not applicable as there is no significant difference.

Finally the authors stated that there was no increase in adverse effects in the lower target diastolic blood pressure groups and that the rate of side effects from medication overall was just 2.2%.

Interpretation: In nondiabetic persons with hypertension, there was no apparent obvious benefit in attempting to achieve a target diastolic blood pressure of 85 mm Hg or 80 mm Hg beyond the benefit achieved by lowering it to 90 mm Hg. In diabetic patients, however, attempting to lower the diastolic pressure to 80 mm Hg resulted in a significant decrease in cardiovascular events, particularly cardiovascular death, with a number needed to treat of just 22. Regarding the aspirin part of the study, hypertensive patients taking low-dose aspirin were less likely to suffer major cardiovascular events, especially myocardial infarction, but the number needed to treat was 200.

Bottom line: The target level for treating blood pressure should be at least to 90 mm Hg, but there is no benefit in striving to get to 85 mm Hg or 80 mm Hg. This conclusion fits with the guideline recommendations of lowering the diastolic blood pressure to <90 mm Hg. For diabetic patients, there is a benefit to lowering the blood pressure to 80 mm Hg. Hypertensive patients benefit from taking low-dose (75 mg) aspirin, but only 1 person would achieve a benefit for every 200 persons taking aspirin.

What did Dr. Sharpe do?

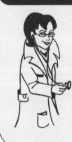

Dr. Sharpe decided to attempt to lower Fitz's blood pressure a bit more. He had a diastolic blood pressure of 92 mm Hg now, so she decided to increase his atenolol dosage to 50 mg daily and recheck him in a month. She also asked him to take 1 "baby" aspirin daily.

Reflection Exercise: How does this evidence apply to your practice? Would you apply this evidence to the management of appropriate patients in your practice? How will your practice change?

Citation: Fodor JG, Frohlich JJ, Genest JJG, McPherson PR, for the Working Group on Hypercholesterolemia and Other Dyslipidemias. Recommendations for the management and treatment of dyslipidemia. Can Med Assoc J 2000; 162:1441–1447.[28]

Validity: This article does not state specific levels of evidence for the recommendations, but it is published by a reputable group and is consistent with recommendations from other agencies and countries.

Table A

Global Risk Assessment Scoring

Patient Name _____

LDL-C _____ TC/HDL _____ TG _____

Diabetes or clinically evident CHD? YES ____ No ____

If YES, at Very High Risk (>30%) proceed to Table B

If No, assess Risk Points

Risk factor		Men	Women	Score
Age(years)	</=34			
	35-39	-1	-9	
	40-44	0	-4	
	45-49	1	0	
	50-54	2	3	___
	55-59	3	6	
	60-64	4	7	
	65-69	5	8	
	70-74	6	8	
Total Cholesterol		7	8	
	</=4.14	-3	-2	
	4.15-5.17	0	0	
	5.18-6.21	1	1	
	6.22-7.24	2	2	___
	>7.24	3	3	
HDL Cholesterol				
	</=0.90		5	
	0.91-1.16	2	2	
	1.17-1.29	1	1	
	1.30-1.66	0	0	___
	>1.55	0	-3	
		-2		
Systolic BP				
	</=120			
	120-129	0	-3	
	130-139	0	0	___
	140-159	1	1	
	>159	2	2	
Smoker		3	3	
	No		0	
	Yes	0	2	___
		2		

TOTAL RISK POINTS →

Table B

Level of Risk	**Target Values**		
(From Table A)	LDL-C	TC/HDL	TG
Very High Risk (10 yr risk >30% or history of CVD or diabetes mellitus)	<2.5	<4.0	<2.0
High Risk (10 yr risk 20-30%)	<3.0	<5.0	<2.0
Moderate Risk (10 yr risk 10-20%)	<4.0	<6.0	<2.0
Low Risk (10 yr risk <10%)	<5.0	<7.0	<3.0

Lipid Targets for this Patient

LDL-C _____ TC/HDL _____ TG _____

Targets Achieved YES ___ No ____

If No   **Treatment**

- Very high or high risk categories (including clinically event CVD or diabetes). If targets not met start medication immediately together with healthy lifestyle modification
- Moderate or low risk categories --- start medication if targets are not met after 3-6 months of healthy lifestyle modification (low- fat high-fibre diet, physical activity, idea body weight, moderate alcohol consumption, smoking cessation)

Medication Choice Based on Major Lipid Abnormality

Lipid Profile	Drug of Choice
Elevated LDL-C	
Alone	Statin +/- resin
+ moderate elev TG	Statin
+ low HDL-C	Statin + fibrate or statin + niacin
Normal LDL-C	
+elevated TG	Niacin or fibrate or combination
+ low HDL-C	Niacin or fibrate

Risk Points →	1	2	3	4	5	6	7	8	9	10	11	12	13	14	15	16	17
10yr CHD Risk For Men→	3%	4%	5%	7%	8%	10%	13%	16%	20%	25%	31%	37%	45%	≥53%			
For Women→	2%	3%	3%	4%	4%	5%	6%	7%	8%	10%	11%	13%	15%	18%	20%	24%	>27%

Fig. 2. Canadian Working Group guidelines on the investigation and treatment of hyperlipidemia.

Cardiovascular risk assessment: Decisions about whether to treat are based on the risk level of the patient. Patients with existing cardiovascular disease or diabetes are classified automatically as high risk and very high risk. For all other patients, a process based on Framingham data is used to calculate risk. This process uses age, total cholesterol, HDL cholesterol, blood pressure, and whether or not the person is a smoker in the assessment of risk level (Fig. 2).

Interpretation: There is an accepted process by which a patient's cardiovascular risk can be assessed, and based on this a decision can be made regarding target levels for lipids and the treatment approach that should be taken.

Bottom line: Treatment decisions should be made based on cardiovascular risk assessment and recommended target levels for lipids.

What did Dr. Sharpe do?

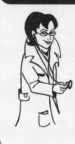

Based on this guideline, Dr. Sharpe decided that Fitz would be classified as very high risk. His recommended target levels would be LDL cholesterol, <2.5 mmol/L; total cholesterol-to-HDL ratio, <4; and triglycerides, <2.0 mmol/L. Fitz has not achieved any of these target levels. Dr. Sharpe increased his simvastatin to 20 mg daily.

Reflection Exercise: How does this evidence apply to your practice? Would you apply this evidence to the management of appropriate patients in your practice? How will your practice change?

Cecilia's Gratitude
(Diabetes Mellitus)

Cecilia is back for her recheck. Her fasting blood glucose today was 8.1 mmol/L, which is better than the 11.8 mmol/L value of 2 weeks ago. After chatting with her about possibly lowering her blood glucose a little more and discussing recognition of hypoglycemic attacks, you increase her glyburide from 5 mg twice daily to 10 mg in the morning and 5 mg in the evening. Cecilia is trained as a nurse, although she hasn't worked in years. Still you are happy that she will be able to recognize and manage hypoglycemia should it occur. You also weigh her.

You check her blood pressure, and it is 140/88 mm Hg, which is good but you recall some recent talk about the target value for blood pressure in diabetics being different than in nondiabetics. You must look into that. For now, you keep her on the ramipril, 10 mg daily, that she is taking.

Cecilia thanks you profusely for not "turning Nick in." When Alexander told her he had received a call from Nick, she was so happy. Just to know he was alive and well, even if he was on the run, was helpful. She also knew that Nick had met with you in Kingston and that he would be calling you again tomorrow. Only she, Alexander, and Joanne knew that Nick had called and that you were involved.

You had a nagging feeling that maybe you shouldn't be involved, but you thought that you now had enough information to convince Nick to give himself up. If Pierre had been having an affair with Amy, there were other possibilities for motives. Still it was a long shot. The finger still pointed more directly at Nick. But perhaps he was tired of hiding.

A question arising from this clinical encounter

25 In a 59-year-old woman with non–insulin-dependent diabetes mellitus and hypertension, does tight control of hypertension decrease the rate of cardiovascular complications of diabetes, and if so, what should the target blood pressure be?

Reflection Exercise:

What are your thoughts regarding this question? Consider this question in the context of your own practice. Consider what you might do before you read the evidence.

Citation: UK Prospective Diabetes Study Group. Tight blood pressure control and risk of macrovascular and microvascular complications in type 2 diabetes: UKPDS 38. BMJ 1998; 317:703–713.[106]

Study design: Randomized controlled trial, blinded, multicentered, with intention-to-treat analysis.

Sample size: 1148

Study population: All participants had hypertension and type 2 diabetes mellitus. They were recruited from 20 hospital-based clinics in England, Scotland, and Northern Ireland. The mean age was 56 years. The mean blood pressure at entry was 160/94 mm Hg.

Intervention group: (N = 758; analyzed = 758): Tight control of blood pressure was attempted with a target blood pressure of <150/85 mm Hg. This group was randomly divided further by using either captopril or atenolol as the main treatment.

Control group: (N = 390; analyzed = 390): Less tight control of blood pressure with a target blood pressure of <180/110 mm Hg but avoiding treatment with either an angiotensin-converting enzyme inhibitor or a β-blocker.

Other study details: Both groups were similar at baseline, including their median fasting blood glucose, which was 7.4 mmol/L in both groups.

The Evidence

Outcome	EER (Tight Blood Pressure Control)	CER (Less Tight Blood Pressure Control)	Relative Risk	ARR	NNTb
Any diabetes-related end point	259 of 758 (34.2%)	170 of 390 (43.6%)	0.76 (0.62–0.92)	9.4%	11
Deaths related to diabetes	82 of 758 (10.8%)	62 of 390 (15.9%)	0.68 (0.49–0.94)	5.1%	20
All-cause mortality	134 of 758 (17.7%)	83 of 390 (21.3%)	0.82 (0.63–1.08)	NA	NA
Myocardial infarction	107 of 758 (14.1%)	69 of 390 (17.7%)	0.79 (0.59–1.07)	NA	NA
Stroke	38 of 758 (5.0%)	34 of 390 (8.7%)	0.56 (0.35–0.89)	3.7%	27
Peripheral vascular disease	8 of 758 (1.0%)	8 of 390 (2.1%)	0.51 (0.19–1.37)	NA	NA
Microvascular disease (retinopathy requiring photocoagulation, vitreous hemorrhage, or renal failure)	68 of 758 (9.0%)	54 of 390 (13.8)	0.63 (0.44–0.89)	4.8%	21

EER, experimental event rate; CER, control event rate; ARR, absolute risk reduction; NNTb, number needed to treat to benefit 1 person; NA, not applicable as there is no significant difference.

Interpretation: This study provides convincing evidence that tighter control of blood pressure in diabetic patients results in lower diabetic complication rates. For every 11 diabetic patients who had their blood pressure better controlled, 1 person did not have a significant adverse outcome that they would have had. If the current guidelines for blood pressure control in diabetics was used (<130/80 mm Hg), these results may have been even better.

Bottom line: Tighter blood pressure control in diabetic hypertensive patients decreases adverse clinical outcomes.

What did Dr. Sharpe do?

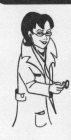

Cecilia's blood pressure was 140/88 mm Hg. This value is not too bad, but the diastolic blood pressure should be lower according to this study (<85 mm Hg). Also the current Canadian guidelines recommend a blood pressure target of <130/80 mm Hg in diabetic patients. So Dr. Sharpe decided to tighten the control of Cecilia's blood pressure. At the next visit, she either will increase the ramipril dosage to 15 mg daily or will add hydrochlorothiazide, 25 mg daily.

Reflection Exercise: How does this evidence apply to your practice? Would you apply this evidence to the management of appropriate patients in your practice? How will your practice change?

Alexander's Quest

(Hypertension)

Alexander was back to have his blood pressure checked and to find out the results of his blood tests. His total cholesterol was down to 6.1 mmol/L, high-density lipoprotein (HDL) was 1.1 mmol/L, low-density lipoprotein (LDL) was 2.8 mmol/L, cholesterol-to-HDL ratio was 5.5, and triglycerides were 2.5 mmol/L. His liver enzymes were normal. His blood pressure today was 150/95 mm Hg. You keep Alex on hydrochlorothiazide, 25 mg daily; start him on ramipril, 5 mg daily; and increase his atorvastatin to 20 mg daily.

It seems that with lipids, lowering cholesterol is the main emphasis for decreasing cardiac risk. You wonder about the importance of triglycerides.

You talk to Alex about his risk of a cardiovascular event given his current risk factors and how much that risk can be decreased. You then ask him how things are at home.

He thanks you for meeting with Nick and for not turning him in. He knows Nick will be calling you later today. He tells you how relieved he was when Nick called him. When he knew Nick was okay, the role of the private investigator who had been hired to find Nick was changed to trying to find out who left Amy Stephens' body in Nick's car and why. Alex thought that the police were focusing on trying to find Nick while the real murderer was being ignored. The private investigator, whose name was Derrick Slade, had discovered some things about Amy (most of which you already knew). Amy had lived with her parents in Bedford until 18 years ago, when they moved to Toronto. She had finished high school, then spent a number of years working as a waitress or barmaid or at other odd jobs. After the abortion episode, she traveled for a year and spent most of the money she had received from Alex. On her return, she went to secretarial school and subsequently worked for a while for a shady group who imported antiques and antiquities from South America. She had dated many different men over the years. One of her recent affairs was with Pierre Savoy.

Alex was angry when he discovered this just yesterday. He had not told Nancy yet but would soon. Pierre was in Toronto on business and would not be returning until Saturday evening. There was going to be a family meeting and confrontation about this. He would talk to Nancy privately first, however.

Slade also had discovered that the affair between Pierre and Amy had ended in February and that Amy had been up to her old tricks again. She had been blackmailing Pierre for $1000 per week, threatening that she would tell Nancy of their affair if he didn't pay. Pierre looked after the financial affairs of much of the Savoy business, so he could hide this money easily from view. Alexander asked you to pass this information on to Nick when he called you later that day and to try to convince him that it was time to go to the police.

A question arising from this clinical encounter

26 In a 60-year-old man with lipid abnormalities involving cholesterol and triglycerides, what is the risk of cardiovascular disease posed by the various components?

_____

Reflection Exercise:

What are your thoughts regarding this question? Consider this question in the context of your own practice. Consider what you might do before you read the evidence.

Answer to Question 26

Citation: Assman G, Cullen P, Schulte H. The Munster Heart Study (PROCAM): Results of follow-up at 8 years. Eur Heart J 1998; 19(Suppl A):A2–A11.[4]

Study design: Cohort study.

Study population: Employees of 52 companies and government authorities. Recruitment phase was completed at the end of 1985. Full records were available for 13,737 men (mean age, 41 ± 11 years) and 5961 women (mean age, 37 ± 12 years). The analysis of major coronary outcomes reported was for a subgroup of 4849 men aged 40–65 years without a prior history of myocardial infarction or stroke and who were followed for 8 years.

Entry data collection: History and physical examination, electrocardiogram, and a 12-hour fasting blood sample for the determination of >20 laboratory parameters, including lipids studies.

Follow-up: Questionnaires sent to participants every 2 years to determine occurrence of myocardial infarction, stroke, or death. Response rate was 96% after two reminders and telephone contact as required. Nonfatal myocardial infarction, fatal myocardial infarction, and cardiac sudden death were defined as major coronary events and were considered end points.

The Evidence: Effect of Total Cholesterol on Occurrence of Any Major Coronary Event over 8 Years

Upper 1/3 of Cholesterol Levels (> 6.2 mmol/L)	Middle 1/3 of Cholesterol Levels (5.3–6.2 mmol/L)	Lower 1/3 of Cholesterol Levels (< 5.3 mmol/L) (Comparison Group)	Relative Risk	ARI	NNEh
142 of 1558 (9.1%)	—	43 of 1505 (2.9%)	3.2 (2.3–4.5)	6.3%	16
—	73 of 1576 (4.6%)	43 of 1505 (2.9%)	1.6 (1.1–2.4)	1.7%	59

ARI, absolute risk increase; NNEh, number needed to be exposed to harm 1 person.

The Evidence: Effect of Low-Density Lipoprotein on Occurrence of Any Major Coronary Event over 8 Years

Upper 1/3 of LDL Levels (>4.2 mmol/L)	Middle 1/3 of LDL Levels (3.4–4.2 mmol/L)	Lower 1/3 of LDL Levels (<3.4 mmol/L) (Comparison Group)	Relative Risk	ARI	NNEh
146 of 1320 (10%)	—	35 of 1521 (2.3%)	4.3 (3.0–6.3)	7.7%	13
—	65 of 1514 (4.2%)	35 of 1521 (2.3%)	1.9 (1.2–3.0)	2%	50

ARI, absolute risk increase; NNEh, number needed to be exposed to harm 1 person.

The Evidence: Effect of High-Density Lipoprotein on Occurrence of Any Major Coronary Event over 8 Years

Lower 1/3 of HDL Levels (<1.0 mmol/L)	Middle 1/3 of HDL Levels (1.0–1.27 mmol/L)	Upper 1/3 of HDL Levels (>1.27mmol/L) (Comparison Group)	Relative Risk	ARI	NNEh
132 of 1582 (8.3%)	—	48 of 1544 (3.1%)	2.7 (1.9–3.8)	5.2%	19
—	78 of 1513 (5.2%)	48 of 1544 (3.1%)	1.7 (1.2–2.4)	2.1%	49

ARI, absolute risk increase; NNEh, number needed to be exposed to harm 1 person.

The Evidence: Effect of Triglycerides on Occurrence of Any Major Coronary Event over 8 Years

Upper 1/3 of Triglyceride Levels (>1.9 mmol/L)	Middle 1/3 of Triglyceride Levels (1.2–1.9 mmol/L)	Lower 1/3 of Triglyceride Levels (<1.2 mmol/L) (Comparison Group)	Relative Risk	ARI	NNEh
128 of 1544 (8.3)	—	48 of 1524 (3.2%)	2.6 (1.9–3.9)	5.1%	19
—	81 of 1571 (5.2%)	48 of 1524 (3.2%)	1.6 (1.1–2.4)	2.0%	50

ARI, absolute risk increase; NNEh, number needed to be exposed to harm 1 person.

All of these effects are independent of each other because even under logistic regression, in which the effect of one factor on the other can be controlled for, the results remained significant for all the lipid factors.

Interpretation: The risk of a major cardiovascular event increases with increasing total cholesterol, LDL, and triglycerides. It also increases with decreasing HDL. Based on absolute risk increases and numbers needed to treat, it would seem that the order of relative importance is LDL, total cholesterol, HDL, and triglycerides. The levels beyond which the risk increases the most dramatically are total cholesterol, >6.2 mmol/L; LDL, >4.2 mmol/L; HDL, <1.0 mmol/L; and triglycerides, >1.9 mmol/L. Because the risk is linear and increases with each unit change in the particular lipid factor, the recommended levels for total cholesterol and LDL tend to be lower than these levels.

Bottom line: All increased values of lipid factors (decreased values for HDL) increase the risk of adverse cardiovascular events. The absolute risk increases of higher levels compared with normal levels are LDL, 7.7%; total cholesterol, 6.3%; HDL, 5.2%; and triglycerides, 5.1%.

What did Dr. Sharpe do?

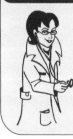

Dr. Sharpe decided that although the various cholesterol components were within reasonable limits, they could be improved, which is why she increased Alex's atorvastatin. She now was more concerned with his triglyceride level and thought that if this did not improve with the increased atorvastatin dosage, she may try a fibrate or niacin.

Reflection Exercise: How does this evidence apply to your practice? Would you apply this evidence to the management of appropriate patients in your practice? How will your practice change?

Joanne's Keys
(Pregnancy)

Joanne was feeling better now that she at least knew Nick was alive, even if he was in hiding. She was feeling fine physically. The nausea and vomiting she had experienced for weeks had settled down. There had been no bleeding and no unusual discharge. You checked the fetal heart and it was 140 beats/min. You talked to her about the VBAC (vaginal birth after cesarean) and the *Gardnerella* and gave her a prescription for oral metronidazole and a requisition to have a urine culture done.

Joanne mentioned that the multivitamin pill she was taking had 3000 IU of vitamin A, and she had heard that it could be bad in pregnancy. You said you would find out the details about this.

Joanne tells you that she knows you have spoken with Nick and that he will be calling you again this evening. She asks you to convince him to go to the police. She knows about the things that Derrick Slade has dug up and thinks the finger can be pointed just as easily away from Nick as toward him.

Joanne also tells you about an episode with her car keys that she thinks is strange but doesn't know if it is related to the case. There were three sets of keys to Nick's dark red BMW—one set that Nick used, one set that Joanne kept in her purse separate from her own keys, and a third spare set that they kept in the house. Joanne and Nancy are close friends. The day before the men had left for Labrador, Nancy had picked Joanne up at her house and they had gone shopping. After a fun day shopping, they stopped at Nancy's on the way home. Joanne was looking for something in her purse and had dumped much of the contents out on the coffee table in the living room. After finding what she was looking for, she collected up all the contents of her purse except for the keys to Nick's car, which she mistakenly left on the table. Nancy drove her home.

The next day the men left for Labrador. Later that same day, Nancy called to tell Joanne that she had left a set of car keys, and they were hanging on one of the key hooks in the kitchen. Joanne didn't get around to picking them up until last week. When she went to get them, Pierre noticed Nancy getting a set of keys off the key hook and said he thought they were his but then seemed to recall something and said no they weren't and apologized. The keys were on a single metal ring without any identification, so it would have been easy to make a mistake.

When Alexander and Pierre had gone back to the Toronto airport to find Nick's car, it had been the third spare set that they kept in the bedroom dresser drawer that Joanne had given them. The police had kept these keys when they confiscated the car. Last week Joanne received a call from the Toronto police saying they had misplaced the keys to the car, the car was locked, and did she have another set. Joanne was annoyed at the seeming incompetence of the police losing the keys but said if they sent someone around to her house she did have another set. This is what prompted Joanne to go to Nancy's finally to pick up the keys she had left there. Shortly after arriving back from Nancy's with the keys, a police officer arrived to pick them up. The next day she received a call from the Toronto police saying the keys had not worked, but they had been able to get into the car using a professional locksmith. They sent her back the keys. She told Nancy about this, and since Nick and Pierre drive the same type of car, they tried the keys in Pierre's dark green BMW and they worked! Pierre had been right when he had said he thought they were his keys. So where were her keys to Nick's car?

You weren't sure how, or if, this story was important to the case but, like Joanne, you thought it was odd.

A question arising from this clinical encounter

27 In a 35-year-old woman who is 13 weeks pregnant, what is the risk to the fetus of taking 3000 IU of vitamin A per day?

Reflection Exercise:

What are your thoughts regarding this question? Consider this question in the context of your own practice. Consider what you might do before you read the evidence.

Answer to Question 27

Citation: Azais-Braesco V, Pascal G. Vitamin A in pregnancy: Requirements and safety limits. Am J Clin Nutr 2000; 71(Suppl):1325S–1333S.[6]

Article type: General review article.

Main Summary Points

1. Vitamin A is an essential micronutrient that plays roles in visual function, growth, reproduction, immunity, and epithelial cell maintenance. Its presence is particularly crucial during periods of rapid cell growth, as in pregnancy and childhood.

2. Vitamin A exerts its functions through oxidized metabolites of retinol.
3. Most vitamin A–dependent functions except for vision can be mediated by retinoic acid.
4. Although low vitamin A status (hypovitaminosis A) in pregnant women has not been related directly to developmental abnormalities, children of these women are vitamin A deficient, and unless they receive sufficient vitamin A after birth, they are at greater risk of morbidity and mortality (diarrhea, respiratory infections, measles).
5. Excessive vitamin A intake leads to acute hypervitaminosis A after the administration of high amounts of the vitamin, usually in a single dose, especially in children.
6. Twenty case reports linked high vitamin A intake in pregnancy and an adverse outcome.
7. Five case-control studies published since 1990 looked at the relationship between supplementation of vitamin A in pregnancy and fetal malformations. In most studies, no association was found between moderate doses of vitamin A (approximately 10,000 IU or 3000 RE) and fetal malformations. In all these studies, the power was low, and so lower dosages also may have teratogenic effect (see table).
8. One prospective study was done that showed doses >10,000 IU (3000 RE) significantly increased the risk of malformations (prevalence ratio, 4.8; 95% confidence interval, 2.2–10.5).
9. One clinical trial was done in Hungary in which supplementation of 6000 IU (1800 RE) of vitamin A did not increase the incidence of fetal malformations. Folic acid was given simultaneously, so it may have interfered with a vitamin A effect on neural tube defects.
10. An adequate vitamin A status, one that is neither too high nor too low, is needed. In industrialized countries, there is no endemicity of low vitamin A status, and consequently there is no need for vitamin A supplementation. Such a measure could be harmful because of the possible teratogenic risk of vitamin A.
11. Over-the-counter supplements ideally should contain low amounts of vitamin A (less than the recommended daily amount). Various countries and agencies have made specific recommendations (see table).

The Evidence: Summary of Case-Control Trials Assessing the Outcome of Fetal Malformation

Cases	Controls	Exposure	Odds Ratio (95% CI)	Comments
11,193	11,293	>10,000 IU/day >40,000 IU/day	1.1 (0.5–2.5) 2.7 (0.8–11.7)	Only 11 cases and 4 controls at the high exposure levels
2658	2609	During 1st month 2nd month 3rd month	2.5 (1.0–6.2) 2.3 (0.9–5.8) 1.6 (0.6–4.5)	No information on vitamin A doses
158	3026	Use of multivitamin supplement	0.57 (0.33–1.00)	Focus on conotruncal defects only
16	12	10,000–14,999 IU/day	1.4 (0.6–2.8)	
426	432	0–9999 IU/day	1	NTDs only; vitamin A from food and supplements
548 NTDs 387 other defects	573	>8000 from supplements	NTDs: 0.91 (0.31–3.68) Other defects: 1.05 (0.51–2.18)	Consumption of liver did not increase risk
		>10,000 from food and supplements	NTDs: 0.73 (0.40–1.53) Other defects: 0.92 (0.40–2.11)	

NTDs, neural tube defects.

The Evidence: Recommendations and Safety Limits of Vitamin A (in IU per Day)

Source	Women Rec	Women SL	Pregnant Women Rec	Pregnant Women SL	Lactating Women Rec	Lactating Women SL	Infants Rec	Infants SL
WHO	500	Low: 270 High: 10,000	600	Low: 450 High: 10,000	850	Low: 450 High: 10,000	350	Low: 180 High: 50,000
U.S.	900	—	900	8000	1350	—	375	—
U.K.	600	—	700	—*	950	—	400	—
France	800	3000	900	3000	1300	3000	350	3000
European Union	600	Low: 250 High: 4000	700	—†	950	—	400	1700

*An official amount not available. †It is stated that "pregnant women on a good diet should not take supplementary vitamin A except under medical advice."

Interpretation: How does one interpret all of this? It seems certain that supplementary vitamin A is not needed in pregnant women who live in developed countries. It is possible that supplemental vitamin A in pregnant women in doses of >10,000 IU/d during the first trimester may cause fetal malformations. The recommended daily amount of vitamin A during pregnancy is generally <1000 IU/d. Most vitamin supplement preparations contain more than this. Although the World Health Organization states that an upper level of safety is 10,000 IU/d, other sources (United States, France) suggest that the safety limit is below this in pregnant women.

Bottom line: There is no need for vitamin A supplementation during pregnancy in women living in developed countries. If supplementation is used, the unsafe level may be 3000 IU/d, and definitely 10,000 IU/d should be avoided.

What did Dr. Sharpe do?

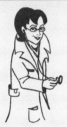

Dr. Sharpe reassured Joanne that the 3000 IU of vitamin A per day she has been taking is unlikely to have caused any problems. She suggested, however, that Joanne use a multivitamin supplement that contains either no vitamin A or <1000 IU and not to take more than one pill per day.

Reflection Exercise: How does this evidence apply to your practice? Would you apply this evidence to the management of appropriate patients in your practice? How will your practice change?

John Hagarty
(Tennis Elbow)

John Hagarty is a 28-year-old carpenter whom you are seeing for the first time. He has developed pain in the lateral aspect of the right elbow. It hurts primarily when he uses his hammer. It is at the point now where it is significantly interfering with his work. On examination, you determine that it is most likely to be tennis elbow and explain it to him.

He says he needs to get this fixed quickly because his boss, the contractor he is working for, is starting to get upset that he is not able to work at his usual capacity. He has a friend who had a similar problem and had it injected. He wonders if that is what he should have done.

A question arising from this clinical encounter

28
In a 28-year-old man with tennis elbow, is local corticosteroid injection effective in reducing pain, and if so, does it work faster than other modalities, such as nonsteroidal anti-inflammatory drugs (NSAIDs) and physical therapy? Does corticosteroid injection have significant potential for complications?

Reflection Exercise:

What are your thoughts regarding this question? Consider this question in the context of your own practice. Consider what you might do before you read the evidence.

Answer to Question 28

Preamble

We found two articles, a systematic review published in 1996 and a randomized controlled trial published in 1999.

Citation: Assendelft WJ, Hay EM, Adshead R, Bouter LM. Corticosteroid injections for lateral epicondylitis: A systematic review. Br J Gen Pract 1996; 46:209–216.[3]

Study design: Systematic review with meta-analysis.

Data sources: Medline 1966–1994, Embase 1980–1994, hand searching of references of relevant articles.

Number of studies: 12

Article selection criteria: Randomized controlled trials; one of the treatments to include one or more corticosteroid injections; patients suffering from epicondylitis; publication in English, German, or Dutch.

Article appraisal process: Methodologic quality was assessed using a standardized criteria list. Factors given various weighting in the assessments were degree of homogeneity, prognostic comparability, handling of dropouts, placebo controls, handling of cointerventions, blinding, and intention-to-treat analysis. Independent assessment was by two different reviewers. Disagreement was resolved by a meeting and consensus. If agreement was not reached, a third reviewer made a final decision.

Data extraction: Outcomes were dichotomized as success or failure and entered into a meta-analysis.

Statistical heterogeneity tests? Yes.

Publication bias resting? No.

Other study details: There was statistical heterogeneity among the studies. The authors decided to pool the data anyway because a large trial is not likely to be done soon.

The Evidence

Outcome	EER*	CER*	Peto Odds Ratio	ARR*	NNTb*
Treatment failure 2–6 weeks post injection	—	—	0.15 (0.10–0.23)	—	—
Treatment failure after 6 weeks post injection	—	—	0.73 (0.37–1.44)	—	—
Treatment failure of "most important follow-up assessment" according to the individual papers' authors	—	—	0.2 (0.12–0.3)	—	—
Treatment failure in the 5 methodologically best studies	—	—	0.14 (0.09–0.23)	—	—
Treatment failure in the 5 methodologically worse studies	—	—	0.49 (0.24–1.02)	—	—

EER, experimental event rate; CER, control event rate; ARR, absolute risk reduction; NNTb, number needed to treat to benefit 1 person.
*The authors did not provide actual numbers to allow us to calculate these factors.

Interpretation: This systematic review seemed to have been done well, but the overall quality of the trials found was low. One major problem with the review was that the absolute outcomes (events) in the studies were not provided, so we are unable to calculate event rates, risk reductions, or numbers needed to treat. From the odds ratios, we can conclude only that the improvement of the epicondylitis was significantly better in the injection groups than in the control groups. In relative terms, it seems to have been a big difference; in absolute terms, we cannot say. This study was repeated in 2002 by the same group. They found one further RCT that they added to the meta-analysis. It did not change the outcome; it still showed only short-term benefits.

Bottom line: Corticosteroid injections may be helpful in the short-term treatment of epicondylitis.

Citation: Hay EM, Oaterson SM, Lewis M, et al. Pragmatic randomized controlled trial of local corticosteroid injection and naproxen for treatment of lateral epicondylitis of elbow in primary care. BMJ 1999; 319:964–968.[39]

Study design: Randomized controlled trial, blinded, multicentered, with intention-to-treat analysis.

Sample size: 164

Study population: Patients from 23 general practices in North Staffordshire and South Cheshire, United Kingdom. There were 164 patients aged 18–70 years presenting with a new episode of lateral epicondylitis.

Intervention group 1: (N = 53; analyzed = 52 or 53): Local injection of 20 mg of methylprednisolone plus 0.5 mL of 1% lidocaine.

Intervention group 2: (N = 53; analyzed = 53): Naproxen, 500 mg twice daily for 2 weeks.

Control group: (N = 58; analyzed = 58 or 56): Placebo tablets.

Outcomes: Outcome measurements were assessed blinded by a study nurse before randomization and at 4 weeks, 6 months, and 12 months. The primary outcome was the patient's global assessment of change measured on a 5-point scale (complete recovery, improved, no change, worse, much worse) at 4 weeks. Secondary outcomes were pain severity, impairment of function, and severity of main complaint, all using a 10-point Likert scale; disability using a disability questionnaire; grip strength using a dynamometer; local tenderness using a 3-point scale; pain on resisted extension of middle finger (3-point scale); number and type of cointerventions; time off paid employment; complications of treatment; local skin atrophy; and gastrointestinal side effects.

Other study details: All patients received a prescription of co-codamol, which is a mixture of acetaminophen and codeine, to use as needed for pain.

The Evidence

Outcome	EER1 (Steroid Injection)	EER2 (Naproxen)	CER (Placebo)	Relative Risk	ABI	NNTb
Complete recovery or some benefit on patient's global assessment of change at 4 wk	48 of 52 (92%)	30 of 53 (57%)	—	1.6 (1.3–1.9)	35%	3
	48 of 53 (92%)	—	28 of 56 (50%)	1.8 (1.4–2.2)	42%	2
		30 of 53 (57%)	28 of 56 (50%)	1.1 (0.8–1.7)	NA	NA
Pain score < 3 out of 10 (at 4 wk)	41 of 53 (82%)	25 of 53 (48%)		1.6 (1.2–2.2)	34%	3
	41 of 53 (82%)		28 of 58 (50%)	1.6 (1.2–2.1)	32%	3
		25 of 53 (48%)	28 of 58 (50%)	0.98 (0.64–1.49)	NA	NA
Pain score < 3 out of 10 (at 6 mo)	33 of 53 (66%)	42 of 53 (81%)		0.78 (0.62–1.03)	NA	NA
	33 of 53 (66%)		47 of 58 (83%)	0.77 (0.61–0.99)	17%*	6*
		42 of 53 (81%)	47 of 58 (83%)	0.98 (0.80–1.19)	NA	NA
Pain score < 3 out of 10 (at 12 mo)	43 of 53 (84%)	45 of 53 (85%)		0.96 (0.80–1.15)	NA	NA
	43 of 53 (84%)		44 of 58 (82%)	1.1 (0.8–1.3)	NA	NA
		45 of 53 (85%)	44 of 58 (82%)	1.1 (0.9–1.3)	NA	NA

EER, experimental event rate; CER, control event rate, ABI, absolute benefit increase; NNTb, number needed to treat to benefit 1 person; NA, not applicable as there is no significant difference.
*These values are for ARI (absolute risk increase) and NNTh (number needed to treat to harm 1 person).

Interpretation: A local steroid injection significantly increases the likelihood that lateral epicondylitis will be improved by 4 weeks compared with using naproxen or placebo. Naproxen was no better than placebo at 4 weeks. By 12 months, regardless of what you do (inject, NSAID, or nothing except pain control), 80–85% of patients are better. If you do nothing but use NSAID or an analgesic, 80–85% of patients are better by 6 months. If you inject a steroid locally, however, there is a greater possibility the pain will flare up again by 6 months. The pain still will have settled by 12 months.

Bottom line: Naproxen works no better than placebo for lateral epicondylitis. Local steroid injections work better than naproxen or placebo at 4 weeks. Patients who receive a local steroid injection may have some increased pain at 6 months compared with naproxen or placebo users. By 12 months, it doesn't matter what you did, 80–85% have resolution of symptoms.

What did Dr. Sharpe do?

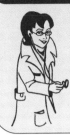

Dr. Sharpe explained the situation to Mr. Hagarty. Because he needs to have relief as soon as possible, he chooses the injection and hopes he is not one of the people who has increased pain after 6 months.

Reflection Exercise: How does this evidence apply to your practice? Would you apply this evidence to the management of appropriate patients in your practice? How will your practice change?

INTERLUDE 2

By 5 PM Friday, you are very tired. It has been a long day, and you still have patient charts to complete. Nick Sampson will be calling at 5:30 PM, and there is so much you have learned since your meeting with him 2 days before—Pierre's recent affair with Amy Stephens and the subsequent blackmail and the men in the dark red BMW, who had met Amy at her house the day she had died. You had also learned that the "secret" about Nick and Amy and her abortion 10 years ago was hardly a secret at all; in fact, everyone seemed to know. What people didn't seem to know about was the money that he and his father had paid to Amy.

You have decided that you would try to convince Nick to turn himself in when he called. There was enough confusion about this case to make the police think of possible killers other than Nick and that was all he said he wanted.

By 5:15 PM, all the staff had left except for Jenny Ling. You noted that Jenny had been around when Nick called the first time. Jenny had an interesting history. She was second-generation Canadian, her parents having come to Canada several years before she was born. Jennifer had worked as the company nurse for the Savoys for many years. The court case that Aunt Joan had mentioned a few days before had ended that employment. Jenny had served as a witness for the employees who were suing the Savoys for unfair employment practices and harassment. Nick Sampson had represented the plaintiffs. The employees had won, Jenny quit her job, and shortly after she was hired to work at the Bedford Family Medicine Clinic. This all had happened before you had arrived in Bedford, but you had chatted with Jenny about it several times.

When the phone rang at 5:30 PM, Jenny answered it immediately and put Nick through to you in your office. You realized then that Jenny must be the other person in the clinic who had been helping Nick. If she hadn't answered the phone within two rings, Nick would have been transferred to the answering system because it was after hours. You had forgotten that, and she knew you would! She obviously had been waiting for the call just like she had been waiting for the first call from Nick a few days earlier. Jenny had been the person who had put that call through to you as well.

You relayed all of your information to Nick. After a little discussion, he agreed to arrive at the clinic at 9 AM tomorrow. The plan was for you to call Fitz, and Nick would call his father. He asked you to arrange with Fitz that they could talk in the clinic as a group before they took him away. You said you would, and after more thanks from Nick you both hung up.

Fitz agreed to the plan.

Jenny was gone when you left the clinic that evening but was unlocking the clinic door at 8:30 AM the next morning when you arrived. It was obvious she was well informed. She put on a pot of coffee while you arranged the chairs in the conference room. At 8:45 AM, Fitz arrived with a police officer from Toronto. At 9:00 AM, another car arrived. Robert Stensen, the Sampson's butler, was driving. In the car was Alexander, Joanne, Derrick Slade, and Nick. They all got out except Robert, who must have been itching to come in to get the scoop. Across the road was a police cruiser with two uniformed policemen watching closely.

The meeting progressed civilly, although it was tense at first. Nick sat by Joanne. She was frightened. Fitz led the meeting. He introduced everyone first, then Nick told his story followed by each person telling what he or she knew. Even though it might be used against him, Nick even told about the payment for the abortion 10 years previously. He had decided to come clean. He also produced the letter that had been sitting on the body bag in his car the evening he arrived back from Labrador.

The police detective from Toronto summarized the case to date, including what had been learned from this meeting:

> Amy Stephens, the victim, had lived in Bedford as a child and teenager but had moved to Toronto with her parents when she was 15 years old. Nick and Amy had met 10 years ago when Amy was 22 and had a one-night stand that resulted in a pregnancy. Amy threatened Nick with a suit for child support but gave him another option. She would have an abortion if Nick paid her $25,000. Nick and Alexander agreed to her demand and paid the $25,000. Nine years later, Pierre Savoy, who is married to Nick's sister, was having an affair with Amy. This affair broke off 4 months before her death. There is evidence though that Amy was up to her old tricks and threatened to tell Pierre's wife unless he paid her $1000 per month. In between these two episodes involving Amy, there was a court case that pitted the Savoys, who were the defendants, against the Sampsons, who defended the plaintiff. The Savoys lost the case and had to pay $100,000. Finally, to complicate matters more, Pierre Savoy married Nancy Sampson after she became pregnant by him.

> This is the story up until the trip to Labrador. Pierre and Nick drive to Toronto in separate cars. The trip apparently goes well. They do go to Labrador; the police have confirmed their stay in a hotel there and have confirmed that they were on the plane back from Labrador on the day Amy was killed. This means neither of them personally could have killed Amy.

> At 1 PM on Thursday, June 22, Amy is picked up at her home by two men driving a dark red BMW. She is killed by strangulation an hour later at 2 PM. At 3 PM, the security cameras show two women arriving in Nick's BMW and leaving in another car that had been parked in the garage.

> Pierre and Nick arrive back in Toronto at 6 PM the same day. Pierre drives away from the parking garage first but doesn't show up at home until midnight. Nick finds the body with the note in his car. He follows the directions in the note, but no one shows up to meet him. He goes into hiding until now.

The police officer goes on to say that there are a number of people who potentially have motives. Nick has a motive because of the previous blackmail episode. The envelope in his car seems to be written to him because the blackmail is alluded to and the $25,000 amount mentioned. Pierre Savoy has a motive because of the ongoing blackmail. There are other more remote possibilities. Maybe Joanne had found out about Nick's past involvement with Amy and wanted her dead. Maybe Pierre's father had noticed the $1000 per month that was missing, found out about the blackmail, and decided to do something about it while Pierre was away. Perhaps Nancy Sampson had uncovered the affair between Pierre and Amy and the ongoing blackmail and decided to do something about it. Maybe Alexander decided he was going to do something about the $25,000 Amy had extracted from him 10 years earlier.

Everyone was quiet as they realized that the police were casting a broad net. No one was beyond doubt. There were many possibilities. None of the scenarios completely explained why the body ended up in Nick's car. The note left in the car sounded as if it were written to Nick and that the person he had hired to kill Amy was now turning the tables on him. But what would Nick's motive be? It seemed odd that he would do this after 10 years. Pierre had a more immediate motive, but nothing else directly implicated Pierre.

Nick was still the number one suspect, and he would have to go with the police to Toronto for further questioning and for a decision as to whether he would be charged. Fitz would be picking up Pierre Savoy for questioning as soon as he arrived back from Toronto later that day.

The meeting ended. Joanne cried as Nick was handcuffed. The two uniformed police came into the clinic and escorted Nick out. The Sampsons followed the police cruiser to Toronto.

The front page of the *Bedford Post* on Monday morning read: PIERRE SAVOY SHOT DEAD IN WAREHOUSE IN TORONTO.

ACT III

Dr. Sharpe's Dilemma
(Gonorrhea)

Nancy Sampson-Savoy did not show up for her appointment at 10 AM, and she had not called to cancel, but you knew why. You had read the details in the newspaper over breakfast. Pierre's body had been found in the Savoy Company warehouse in Toronto. He had been shot twice in the head. Police were looking for a suspect named Leo Nash. The paper also reported that the police believed there might be a connection between this murder and the murder of Amy Stephens 2 weeks earlier.

You decided to call Nancy to see how she was. You also had some further bad news for her that you did not want to have to deal with. Her cervical cultures were positive for gonorrhea. This woman who had just lost her husband may not know yet that he had recently been unfaithful to her. You now had to tell her that his unfaithfulness had led to her contracting gonorrhea. She also would have to be screened for HIV and hepatitis B and C.

You still hadn't decided what to do as you dialed the number. There was no answer at her house, but you realized immediately there wouldn't be. She was probably at her parents' home. You dialed Alexander and Cecilia's number. Alexander answered the phone. As soon as he realized who it was, he asked you not to mention Pierre's infidelity to Nancy. They had not told her, and with the news of Pierre's death, they decided it was best not to tell her now. You reminded him that these details were likely to come out if there was ever a trial, and he said he knew that, but for now he thought it would be too much for Nancy to bear. You said you understood and that you would not mention it to Nancy, but you would like to speak to her if you could.

When Nancy came to the phone, you could tell from her voice she had been crying. You offered your condolences and asked if there was anything you could do. She thanked you for your call, apologized for not keeping her appointment this morning, and said that she would come in later. You told her not to worry about missing the appointment and to come in whenever she wished. You were just about to hang up when she asked if the cultures were back yet. You hesitated for a minute, said they were not, but that they would be soon and she should come in next week.

This was a real problem! Nancy was bound to find out sooner or later. Either it would come out in the trial, or she would get active gonorrhea. Later that day, the Health Unit called saying they had received a copy of the positive result and asked if you were going to treat, screen for other sexually transmitted diseases (STDs), and follow up contacts. You said you would. There was no getting out of this one. Next week, at the latest, you would have to break the news to Nancy. You wondered if waiting that long was putting her at risk.

Some questions arising from this clinical encounter

29 In a 30-year-old woman with culture-positive, asymptomatic gonorrhea, what is the likelihood of progression to active clinical disease over a 1-week period?

30 In a 30-year-old woman with gonorrhea, what is the likelihood that she also has contracted HIV or hepatitis?

Reflection Exercise:

What are your thoughts regarding these questions? Consider them in the context of your own practice. Consider what you might do before you read the evidence.

Answer to Question 29

Preamble

We did not find an article that directly answers this question in an evidence-based manner. We report here on two sources of information.

Citation: Sparling PF. Gonococcal infections. In: Cecil's Textbook of Internal Medicine. MDConsult available at http://www.mdconsult.com.[99]

Document type: Chapter in a medical textbook.

Points pertinent to clinical question:
1. Approximately 50% of women infected with *Gonococcus* are asymptomatic or have so few symptoms that they do not seek medical care.
2. About 15% of women with gonococcal cervicitis develop pelvic inflammatory disease (PID).
3. The time frame from contracting gonococcal cervicitis to PID is not given.

Citation: Centers for Disease Control and Prevention. 1998 Guidelines for treatment of sexually transmitted diseases. MMWR Morbid Mortal Wkly Rep 1998; 47:1–111.[16]

Document type: Guideline.

Pertinent points:
1. Many infections among women do not produce recognizable symptoms until complications (PID) have occurred.
2. Women at high risk for STDs should be screened.

Interpretation: There is not enough information to answer this question precisely. It seems, however, that only 15% of women who have gonococcal infection develop PID. The time frame between when a gonococcal infection is contracted and when PID occurs is not stated. It seems that the risk can be substantial.

What did Dr. Sharpe do?

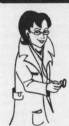

Dr. Sharpe decided that given the limited information she had and given the current situation, she would wait at least a few more days before telling Nancy the news and starting treatment. Sometimes decisions in medicine have to be made on limited information and considering the patient's circumstances.

Reflection Exercise: How does this evidence apply to your practice? Would you apply this evidence to the management of appropriate patients in your practice? How will your practice change?

Answer to Question 30

Citation: Torian LV, Makki HA, Menzies IB, et al. High HIV seroprevalence associated with gonorrhea: New York City Department of Health, sexually transmitted disease clinics, 1990–1997. AIDS 2000; 14:189–195.[103]

Study design: Unlinked HIV-1 serosurvey using serum originally drawn for routine serologic tests for syphilis.

Study population: Data were collected between 1990 and 1997. The serosurveys were conducted during 4–6 month periods in five sentinel STD clinics. Patients were eligible if the visit was for a new episode of illness, if they had not visited the clinic in 90 days, and if they had not presented just for HIV testing. This led to a sample of 1200–2000 patients per clinic per year.

Data collection: Serum that had been collected for syphilis testing was used for HIV testing. Other STD testing was done, including cultures for gonococcal infection.

The evidence: HIV seroprevalence in patients diagnosed with gonorrhea remained steady at 10–11% throughout 1990–1997. Seroprevalence for all other STDs declined from 8% to 5% during the same period.

Interpretation: Patients with gonorrhea have about a 10% likelihood of also being positive for HIV in New York City.

Bottom line: Of people with gonorrhea, 10% are also HIV-positive.

> Citation: Hershow RC, Kalish LA, Sha B, et al. Hepatitis C virus infection in Chicago women with or at risk for HIV infection. Sexual Transm Dis 1998; 527–532.[43]

Study design: Cross-sectional study.

Study population: Chicago women newly enrolled in the Women's Interagency HIV Study. Women who had HIV infection (N = 243) or were at risk for HIV infection (N = 53) were tested for hepatitis C virus antibodies. Total sample was 296.

The evidence: Of 296 women, 123 (42%) were hepatitis C virus positive.

Interpretation: In a large city population of women with HIV or at high risk of HIV, there is a 42% prevalence of hepatitis C infection.

Bottom line: Prevalence of hepatitis C virus in HIV-positive patients is 42%.

What did Dr. Sharpe do?

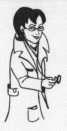

Dr. Sharpe realized she would have to screen Nancy for HIV and hepatitis C. The evidence of a 10% association with HIV and 5% association with other STDs is primarily for an inner-city population in the United States. If Nancy contracted the STD from her husband, Pierre, who had contracted it from Amy Stephens, who probably had had many Toronto inner-city contacts, the data might apply to her.

Reflection Exercise: How does this evidence apply to your practice? Would you apply this evidence to the management of appropriate patients in your practice? How will your practice change?

Fitz's Worst Fear

(Angina)

Fitz came to see you in an uncharacteristic agitated mood. During his 5-km walk the evening before, he had noticed a little tightness in his chest. He felt a similar episode this morning while showering. It had been 2 years since his coronary artery bypass graft (CABG) surgery, and this was the first time he had felt that sensation since before the operation. His father and grandfather had died in their 50s of heart disease, and Fitz was, to be honest, terrified.

You took a detailed history. He had walked about 2 km last evening when the tightness started. He slowed down immediately, then stopped and sat on a bench. The tightness went away after a couple of minutes. He didn't have any nitroglycerin on him because it had been so long since he'd needed it he didn't carry it anymore. The tightness was not associated with any weakness, sweating, nausea, or shortness of breath. He had no sensation in his arm or jaw. This morning the tightness was exactly the same during his shower.

On examination, his blood pressure was 150/94 mm Hg, and his pulse was 64 beats/min. His chest was clear, and his heart sounds were normal. There was no pedal edema.

You call his cardiologist, who suggests you add long-acting nitroglycerin to his medication regimen and make sure he has nitroglycerin spray with him all the time. He will see Fitz in a week. If there are signs of increasing or prolonged pain, however, he is to go to the emergency department immediately. You wonder what this means prognostically for Fitz.

Fitz is happy with the plan. He doesn't ask any questions about what it means for him if this is a recurrence of angina, but you suspect that is because he doesn't want to know right now.

You ask how things are going with the investigation. Fitz tells you about how they had been waiting outside Pierre Savoy's home on Saturday evening to pick him up for questioning when he returned from Toronto, but he never arrived. At 11 PM, they had knocked on the door to see if he had arrived back without them seeing him. Nancy had answered the door, and they explained that they wanted to speak with Pierre. She said he wasn't home, but that she had been expecting him hours earlier and was getting worried. Fitz informed the Toronto police of the situation, and they put an alert out for him. It wasn't until late on Sunday afternoon that his body was found by the supervisor of the Savoy Company's Toronto warehouse, who had gone there on a routine check.

Pierre had been shot twice in the head on Saturday afternoon. There was no evidence of breaking and entry. There was no evidence of theft.

You suggested that Fitz take the rest of the week off until he saw the cardiologist. He said he would try but couldn't promise to take time completely off work because he had a lot of backed-up paperwork. He did promise to contact you or go to the emergency department if the pain recurred.

A question arising from this clinical encounter

31

In a 53-year-old man who develops recurrence of chest pain 2 years after successful CABG surgery, what is the 5-year survival and the likelihood of further surgery being required?

Reflection Exercise:

What are your thoughts regarding this question? Consider this question in the context of your own practice. Consider what you might do before you read the evidence.

Answer to Question 31

Preamble

Outcomes and predictors after CABG surgery have been well studied. We present four articles here.

Citation: Herlitz J, Brandrup-Wognsen G, Karlson BW, et al. Mortality, risk indicators of death, mode of death and symptoms of angina pectoris during 5 years after coronary artery bypass grafting in men and women. J Intern Med 2000; 247:500–506.[42]

Study design: Prospective follow-up cohort of CABG surgery patients.

Study population: Patients (2365) undergoing CABG surgery between 1988 and 1991 in western Sweden. Patients were excluded if they had concomitant valve procedures or if they had had previous CABG surgery. After these exclusions, there was a sample size of 2000, of which 381 (19%) were women. They were followed for 5 years.

The evidence:
1. In men, 5-year mortality rate was 13.3%.
2. In women, 5-year mortality rate was 17.3%, which was significantly higher (relative risk, 1.4; 95% confidence interval, 1.0–1.8). Women were at higher risk at baseline, however, and after adjusting for these differences, the risk of death was the same as men.
3. Congestive heart failure and diabetes mellitus were independent risk factors for death in men and women.
4. At 5 years, women had substantially more symptoms of angina pectoris than men.

Interpretation: The 5-year mortality rate after CABG surgery is about 13.3%.

Bottom line: The 5-year mortality rate after CABG surgery is about 13.3%.

Citation: Skinner JS, Farrer M, Albers CJ, et al. Patient-related outcomes five years after coronary artery bypass graft surgery. QJM 1999; 92:87–96.[97]

Study design: Prospective follow-up cohort study.

Study population: Patients (353) undergoing CABG surgery between October 1988 and December 1989 were followed prospectively for 5 years. There were 297 men and 56 women. Mean age was 57 (SD 7) years.

The Evidence: Outcomes 5 Years Post Coronary Artery Bypass Graft Surgery

Outcomes	No. (%)
Death over 5 y	41 (12%)
Angina	
Pre-CABG	Nearly 100%
3 mo	16%
6 mo	28%
12 mo	30%
60 mo	45%
Employed (working)	
Pre-CABG	123 (36%)
3 mo	44 (14%)
6 mo	98 (32%)
12 mo	104 (34%)
60 mo	60 (21%)

CABG, coronary artery bypass graft.

Interpretation: The rate of return of angina after surgery shows a steady increase, such that at 5 years 45% of patients again have angina symptoms. The death rate over 5 years is 12%.

Bottom line: By 5 years post–CABG surgery, 12% of patients are dead, and nearly half of the remaining have angina.

Citation: Chan AW, Ross J. Management of unstable coronary syndromes in patients with previous coronary artery bypass grafts following coronary angiography. Clin Invest Med 1997; 20:320–326.[17]

Study design: Descriptive retrospective study.

Study population: Patients (129) with one previous (CABG) procedure who underwent coronary angiography for myocardial infarction or unstable angina in 1991.

Outcome measures: Early complications and 1-year outcomes of patients using three treatment modalities: drugs, angioplasty, or repeat CABG surgery.

The Evidence

Early Complications	Drug Therapy (n = 76)	Angioplasty (n = 28)	Repeat CABG (n = 25)
Death	4 (5.3%)	0	1 (4%)
Nonfatal myocardial infarction	1 (1.3%)	1 (4%)	2 (8%)
Nonfatal ventricular arrhythmia	8 (11%)	1 (4%)	11 (44%)
Procedure-related complications	NA	7 (25%)	7 (28%)

CABG, coronary artery bypass graft; NA, not applicable as there is no significant difference.

The Evidence

Outcomes at 1 Year	Drug Therapy (47 Available for Follow-up)	Angioplasty (24 Available for Follow-up)	Repeat CABG (16 Available for Follow-up)
Death	3 (6.4%)	0	0
Repeat angioplasty	3 (6.4%)	12 (50%)	0
Repeat CABG	2 (4.3%)	2 (8.3%)	0
Recurrent angina	14 (30%)	15 (63%)	3 (19%)
Improvement of >2 classes (Canadian Cardiovascular Society Classification)	9 (19%)	5 (21%)	8 (50%)

CABG, coronary artery bypass graft.

Interpretation: This study looks at patients who have had a CABG procedure previously and now have a return of symptoms in whom angiography is performed and a decision about treatment is made. Generally, in patients in whom the decision is made to treat surgically (angioplasty or CABG surgery), there are better outcomes from the perspective of survival and symptom improvement.

Bottom line: Patients who require angiography and a treatment decision after having had a previous CABG procedure generally tend to have a complicated course. Patients who undergo another surgical procedure (angioplasty or CABG surgery) seem to do better, however.

Citation: Kaul TK, Fields BL, Riggins LS, et al. Reinterventions for recurrent ischemic heart disease following a successful first re-do myocardial revascularization: predictors, indications and results. Cardiovasc Surg 1999; 7:363–369.[53]

Study design: Follow-up cohort study.

Study population: Patients (302) who previously had had a redo surgical revascularization and who now required a further intervention. Of patients, 158 (52%) had graft angioplasty and 114 (48%) had redo CABG surgery.

Time frame: 1988–1995.

The Evidence

Outcome	Graft Angioplasty	Redo CABG
Cardiac events (further procedures, myocardial infarction and death)		
After 1 mo	20%	5.5%
After 1 y	40.5%	10%
After 8 y	66%	56.5%
Actuarial survival at 6 y	77%	83%

CABG, coronary artery bypass graft.

Interpretation: This study looks at the results of a third major intervention. Redo CABG surgery seems to be a better choice than angioplasty of the previous graft that has become occluded.

Bottom line: CABG surgery is a better choice than angioplasty for the third intervention for coronary artery stenosis.

Overall summary: The 5-year mortality rate in men who have had CABG surgery is about 12–13%. Approximately 45% have recurrent angina, and about 21% still work at their job after 5 years. If a person with previous CABG surgery develops unstable angina or a myocardial infarction, there are three main treatment options: drugs, redo CABG surgery, or angioplasty. The 1-year outcomes seem to be better if a surgical approach (redo CABG surgery or graft angioplasty) is chosen. Only 1 of 25 (4%) patients was dead after 1 year in the redo surgical groups, whereas 7 of 76 (9%) patients were dead in the drug treatment group. Because these are all observational studies and not randomized trials, the effects of different treatments may not be completely accurate. Patients with more severe and inoperable coronary artery stenosis may have been given drug treatment, whereas patients more likely to survive may have been operated on.

What did Dr. Sharpe do?

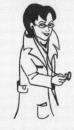

Given the results of these studies, Dr. Sharpe decided that although Fitz's likelihood of surviving 5 years immediately after the CABG procedure had been done was about 88%, this probably no longer was the case now that his angina had recurred. The success rate of a redo CABG procedure seemed good, however, at least according to the 1-year survival rates for redo CABG procedures. Dr. Sharpe thought the odds were reasonable for Fitz, and if the surgeon and cardiologist suggested a redo procedure, Fitz should be encouraged to have it done as opposed to just using medications.

Reflection Exercise: How does this evidence apply to your practice? Would you apply this evidence to the management of appropriate patients in your practice? How will your practice change?

Robert's Connections
(Testicular Lump)

Robert Stensen was the butler and driver for the Sampson family. Stefan Richard had a similar position with the Savoy family. It was no secret that Robert and Stefan were lovers. Their employers knew and accepted it. You had heard Alexander say many times how he relied on Robert for many things and that what Robert did on his own time was his business.

There wasn't much of a gay community in Bedford, at least not a freely open one. Robert and Stefan went to Toronto on their days off together. The gay community there was open in that gays did not hide who and what they were, but at the same time the community was tight. Secrets were kept. Things were known. Often members of the gay community knew more about the underbelly of Toronto society than the police did. Everyone knew Leo Nash and his sidekick Joey Hynes. Joey was gay, and Leo was bisexual. Leo was a bit of a scumbag and a lowlife. He had been in jail for breaking and entry, but most of the crimes he had committed had gone unpunished. He had even been used at times by organized crime to help persuade some people to see things "the right way" and to make people "disappear."

The buzz around the gay scene was that Leo had been hired to kill Amy Stephens. Apparently Amy had been blackmailing Pierre Savoy for months, and a few weeks before her death she had increased the blackmail amount, from $1000 per week to $2000 per week some said. It was generally thought that Pierre had hired Leo to kill Amy. What nobody could figure out was who killed Pierre, unless Leo had done that as well.

Robert talked to you about this before he even mentioned what he was in to see you about. Robert loved to talk. So did Stefan. If the Sampsons and Savoys only knew what they told their doctor! You suspected that Robert knew the amounts of the blackmail because Stefan had checked the financial records of the Savoys. Robert would never say that, of course, because it would implicate Stefan in a crime. They were loyal and never told stories about each other.

Robert was in because he had a lump in his testicle. It wasn't painful or sore. He had no problems voiding or with sexual intercourse. Stefan had noticed it first about 2 months ago. Robert had checked it daily since then and wasn't certain if it had changed in size.

On examination, the lump was about 1 cm and in the midportion of the left testicle. It appeared to be fixed and not mobile. There was no redness or tenderness. There were no grain nodes. The prostate was normal. The other testicle was normal.

Robert was worried. He asked if you thought it was cancer or a sexually transmitted disease. You told him you were fairly certain it wasn't a sexually transmitted disease. You couldn't say with certainty, however, whether it was anything to worry about. You told him that benign cysts were common but that to be sure you would arrange an ultrasound and a referral to a urologist.

After Robert left, you called Fitz and told him about the two guys, Leo Nash and Joey Hynes, that Robert had mentioned. You didn't know whether it would be useful, but you thought it was at least worth letting the police know. The worse that could happen is that it would be a false lead to nowhere.

Some questions arising from this clinical encounter

32 In a 35-year-old man with a 1-cm testicular lump, what is the most likely diagnosis, and which factors affect prognosis?

33 In a 35-year-old man with a 1-cm testicular lump, how useful is ultrasound in ruling out cancer?

Reflection Exercise:

What are your thoughts regarding these questions? Consider them in the context of your own practice. Consider what you might do before you read the evidence.

Answer to Question 32

Citation: Macksood MJ, James RE. The scrotal mass: Cause and diagnosis. Am J Surg 1983; 145:297–299.[65]

Study design: Retrospective chart review.

Study population: Patients (278) who presented with either a painful or an asymptomatic scrotal or testicular mass during the 7-year period from January 1974 to December 1980. Patients with inguinal hernia or hydrocele associated with inguinal hernia were not included.

The Evidence: Causes of Scrotal Masses in 278 Patients

Cause of mass	No. (%)
Inflammatory masses	133 (48)
Hydrocele	66 (24)
Testicular torsion	20 (7)
Varicocele	19 (7)
Spermatocele	12 (4)
Various cysts	11 (4)
Malignant tumors	6 (2)
Benign tumors	2 (1)
Others	9 (3)

Interpretation: The likelihood of a scrotal mass being malignant is low (2%). The likelihood of malignancy if the mass is definitely in the testicle itself may be higher. This study does not differentiate between these two situations.

Bottom line: Scrotal masses in general are usually benign.

Citation: Walsh. Campbell's Urology. 7th edition. Philadelphia: WB Saunders; p. 143.[109]

The authors of this book state, without referring to a source: "A useful guideline is that most masses arising from the testicle are malignant, whereas almost all masses arising from the spermatic cord structures are benign."

Citation: Townsend. Sabiston Textbook of Surgery. 16th edition. Philadelphia: WB Saunders; p. 1690.[104]

The authors of this book state, without referring to a source: "Testicular cancer, although relatively rare, represents the most common malignancy in males in the 15- to 35-year-old age group. It has become one of the most curable solid neoplasms and serves as a paradigm for the multimodal treatment of malignancies."

Citation: Mostofi FK. Testicular tumors: Epidemiologic, etiologic, and pathologic features. Cancer 1973; 32:1186–1201.[71]

This study is referred to frequently in the urologic literature. It is primarily a histologic study.

Study design: Retrospective review of 7000 testicular tumors registered in the Testicular Tumor Registry of the American Urological Association.

The evidence:
1. Incidence, 2.1–2.2 per 100,000 males per year.
2. Testicular cancer is the fourth most common cause of cancer death in ages 15–34 years (note that this is "cause of cancer death," not incidence of cancer; in a previous citation, testicular cancer was said to be the most common cancer in this age group).

Summary: It seems that cancer of the testicle is uncommon, but men in their 20s and 30s are the most likely to develop it. A mass in the testicle itself, as opposed to the supporting structures, makes it more likely that a malignancy is present.

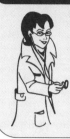

What did Dr. Sharpe do?

Dr. Sharpe had referred Robert to a urologist. Now, reflecting on the results of her literature review, that seemed to have been the correct choice. Even though the direct evidence on which it was claimed that masses in the testicle itself were more likely to be cancer was not apparent, this seemed to be a consensus.

Reflection Exercise: How does this evidence apply to your practice? Would you apply this evidence to the management of appropriate patients in your practice? How will your practice change?

Answer to Question 33

Citation: Polak V, Hornak M. The value of scrotal ultrasound in patients with suspected testicular tumour. Int Urol Nephrol 1990; 20:467–473.[82]

Study design: A prospective study of 56 patients with suspected testicular tumor. The suspicion of testicular tumor was raised based on examination of scrotal contents.

Study population: Age range was 2–67 years (mean, 26 years). Study was conducted in Czechoslovakia, 1986–1989.

Data collection: All patients had ultrasound of the scrotal contents, and the results were correlated with findings at time of surgery.

The Evidence

	Tumor at Surgery		
	Yes	No	
Ultrasound Positive	35	8	43
Negative	2	11	13
	37	19	56

		95% Confidence Intervals
Sensitivity	95%	87–100
Specificity	58%	36–80
Positive predictive value	81%	70–93
Negative predictive value	85%	65–100
Positive likelihood ratio	2.25	1.32–3.83
Negative likelihood ratio	0.09	0.02–0.38

Interpretation: Ultrasound is a SnNout for testicular cancer. Because the test is highly sensitive (Sn), if it is negative (N), it rules the condition out. This is proved in the negative likelihood ratio, which tells us that the likelihood of cancer is reduced considerably if the ultrasound if negative. A negative likelihood ratio of 0.09 means the posttest probability of its being cancer is only 10% that of the pretest probability. If the test is positive, however, you still cannot be certain it is cancer because the specificity is only 58%. There are a significant number of false-positive results.

Bottom line: A negative ultrasound is useful at ruling out cancer in patients presenting with scrotal masses.

What did Dr. Sharpe do?

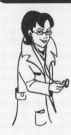

Dr. Sharpe was glad she had requested an ultrasound. Perhaps she had acted too quickly, however, in suggesting she also would arrange an appointment with a urologist. If the ultrasound was negative, it was unlikely to be cancer. She decided she would discuss it further with Robert when he returned and perhaps just call a urologist when she got the results of the ultrasound.

Reflection Exercise: How does this evidence apply to your practice? Would you apply this evidence to the management of appropriate patients in your practice? How will your practice change?

Gemma and Her Dad
(Urinary Tract Infection and Colorblindness)

Gemma was a cute little blond girl. Her father brought her in because her mother, who was a nurse, was working, and Mr. Simms had more flexibility in his schedule. He had his own business, a milk packager and distributor, and was able to take time off more easily.

Gemma had been crying and "complaining" of pain in the vulvar area for a couple of days. They had used some clotrimazole cream first, but it hadn't helped. She hadn't seemed sick or feverish at any time. She cried when she used her potty. On examination, her vulva was red, but you didn't notice anything to suggest trauma. Mrs. Simms, anticipating that you might want to check her urine, had managed to collect some using an adhesive urine collection bag. It was collected last night so might have been hours old.

You checked the urine with a dipstick and microscope. There were lots of bacteria, but that was to be expected given the means of collection and the fact that it had been lying around at body temperature for a while. There was also blood, which might have been due to the irritated vulva, and many white cells. The white cells also could be due to the vulvitis. The dipstick test for nitrates was negative.

You arrange to have another urine sample collected using an adhesive collection bag and ask Mr. Simms to make sure it is collected in the daytime and to check it frequently so that as soon as she has voided the specimen is brought into the laboratory. You explain to Mr. Simms that Gemma will have to see a pediatrician and may need a cystoureterogram done. It all sounds very invasive to the father, and he asks why the infection simply can't be treated and see what happens.

Just before leaving, Mr. Simms mentions that he will be in later to have a physical for a driver's license. He wants to be licensed to drive their large truck. His brother has done all the truck driving to date. Mr. Simms mentions that he thinks he is possibly colorblind but has never been tested for it.

34 In an 18-month-old girl with symptoms suggestive of a urinary tract infection (UTI), how useful is the nitrate dipstick test for ruling in or ruling out significant bacteriuria?

35 In an 18-month-old girl with symptoms suggestive of a UTI, how accurate is a specimen collected by an adhesive collector on the perineum?

36 In an 18-month-old girl with a confirmed UTI, what is the likelihood of serious complications if the child is treated for each clinically apparent infection without having invasive urologic investigations carried out?

37 In a 30-year-old man, how would colorblindness affect his ability to drive?

Reflection Exercise:

What are your thoughts regarding these questions? Consider them in the context of your own practice. Consider what you might do before you read the evidence.

Answer to Question 34

Citation: Gorelick MH, Shaw KN. Screening tests for urinary tract infection in children: A meta-analysis. Pediatrics 1999; 104:1–7.[32]

Study design: Systematic review with meta-analysis.

Data sources: Medline.

Number of studies: 26

Number of patients: 1868

Time frame: 1975–1998

Article selection criteria: Primary data only, results of dipstick or microscopic urinalysis compared with urine culture.

Details: The study used a nonstandard approach to presenting the results such that it was not always easy to determine the sensitivity, specificity, and likelihood ratios for the various tests. For certain tests, the likelihood ratios are stated directly and are given in the table.

The Evidence

Test	LR +ve	LR −ve
Gram stain	18.5	0.07
Leukocytes and nitrites	12.6	0.13
Nitrites only	14.4	0.27
Bacteria on Gram stain and ≥10 WBCs	85	0.06

LR +ve, likelihood ratio for a positive test; LR −ve, likelihood ratio for a negative test; WBCs, white blood cells.

Interpretation: A rough interpretation is if a Gram stain is positive, the posttest likelihood that a UTI exists is 18.5 that of the likelihood an infection existed before the test results were known. A positive Gram stain makes it highly likely that an infection exists. If a Gram stain is negative, the posttest likelihood that a UTI exists is 7/100, or 1/14th that of the likelihood an infection existed before the test result was known. A negative Gram stain makes it highly likely that an infection does not exist. The same interpretation can be applied to the leukocytes and nitrites and the combination of Gram stain and white blood cell count.

The results for nitrites alone were more difficult to discern from this article and are only approximations. They suggest, however, that a positive result is good at ruling in an infection (positive likelihood ratio of 14.4), whereas a negative results is less reliable for ruling out an infection (negative likelihood ratio of 0.27).

Bottom line: A positive dipstick test for nitrites rules in a UTI. If it is negative it makes a UTI less likely, but it cannot be relied on with certainty for the diagnosis.

What did Dr. Sharpe do?

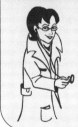

Dr. Sharpe strongly suspected a UTI based on the history. She could not rely on the negative nitrites test. She arranged for a repeat urine specimen for culture.

Reflection Exercise: How does this evidence apply to your practice? Would you apply this evidence to the management of appropriate patients in your practice? How will your practice change?

Answer to Question 35

Citation: Liaw LCT, Nayar DM, Pedler SJ, Coulthard MG. Home collection of urine for culture from infants by three methods: Survey of parents' preferences and bacterial contamination rates. BMJ 2000; 320:1312–1313.[63]

Study design: Prospective study.

Study population: Forty-four children age 1–18 months with no symptoms of UTI and their parents.

Study details: Parents were asked to collect three urine samples from their child using three different methods: pads, bags, and clean catch. Parents were asked to rate their preference of methods. Cultures were rated as no significant growth, contamination, or positive (see criteria in Table).

The Evidence

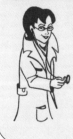

	No Significant Growth ($< 10^4$/ml)	Contamination ($> 10^4$/ml)	Infection (10^5/ml)	Unable to Collect
Pad	31 (70%)	7 (16%)	4 (9%)	2 (5%)
Bag	29 (66%)	8 (18%)	5 (11%)	2 (5%)
Clean catch	33 (75%)	2 (5%)	0	9 (20%)

In order of preference of method, parents liked the pads best, then the bag, and the clean-catch method least of all. In two children, no samples were collected: one had diarrhea, and the other had a UTI. In seven other children, the parents gave up on trying to get a clean-catch specimen, finding it too long and frustrating.

Note: In two other studies,[18,62] similar results were found. In one of these studies, the pad was identical to catheter or suprapubic tap for positive and negative results. The authors of these trials thought the pad could be used instead of invasive methods.

Interpretation: The concern with pads and bags for collecting urine specimens in children is that they give a high false-positive rate. This study shows that the false-positive rates for these methods are only in the range of 10%. If urine specimens collected by these methods are negative for infection, you can be fairly certain there is no infection. If the urine specimen is positive for infection, further testing should be done to confirm. If this process were applied, it would decrease the need for collection of specimens by suprapubic needle aspiration.

Bottom line: A negative culture by pad or bag rules out UTI. A positive culture may require that further testing be done.

What did Dr. Sharpe do?

Dr. Sharpe asked Gemma's dad to collect another urine specimen using a bag. If it is negative, she will feel confident there is no infection. If the specimen is positive, she will ask the pediatric urologist for advice about further culture techniques. She disliked having to do suprapubic aspirations or catheterizations in children. She may just treat if a UTI is suggested by the bag collection.

Reflection Exercise: How does this evidence apply to your practice? Would you apply this evidence to the management of appropriate patients in your practice? How will your practice change?

Citation: Dick PT, Feldman W. Routine diagnostic imaging for childhood urinary tract infections: A systematic review. J Pediatr 1996; 128:15–22.[22]

Study design: Systematic review.

Data sources: Medline, Current Contents, scanning of reference lists of articles.

Number of studies: 434 found; 63 met criteria; 9 prospective used.

Number of patients: 1219

Time frame: 1966–1994

Article selection criteria: Controlled trials, analytic case-control or controlled cohort studies, descriptive studies. The primary medical subject headings used to search were *pyelonephritis* and *vesicoureteral reflux.* Case series based on urologic anomalies or including adults were excluded. Editorials, commentaries, and reviews were excluded as were articles exclusively regarding neonatal UTIs or asymptomatic bacteriuria. Multiple other search strategies were used to ensure that important articles were not missed.

Article appraisal process: A random sample of the articles was reviewed by both authors to determine interrater reliability. There was 100% interrater agreement on inclusion eligibility and design classification and excellent agreement on sample selection categories (κ 0.81).

Other study details: The main search strategy yielded 434 articles, of which 63 met the inclusion criteria. No controlled trials or analytic studies evaluating or comparing different management strategies were discovered. All studies were descriptive in design, and most sampled children through referral for consultation, radiologic investigation, hospitalization, or recurrent UTIs. Of the 63 studies, only 9 used prospective recruitment of cases with specific inclusion criteria. No studies described exclusively first UTIs in a primary care setting. Only the 9 studies were used for formal analysis. A meta-analysis was not done because all studies were descriptive.

The Evidence: Abnormalities Present on Imaging at Time of Diagnosis

Study	Inclusion Criteria	Diagnostic Imaging	Vesicoureteral Reflux	Radiographic Obstruction	Renal Scarring on Presentation
Rosenberg (1992)	1st UTI, 69% <4 y	RI/IVP, US, ± VCUG	24.4%	—	—
Tappin (1989)	1st UTI, birth to 14 y	RI, VCUG, ± US	29%	4%	—
Pylkkannen (1981)	1st UTI, birth to 14 y	IVP ± VCUG	8%	0.8%	—
Hellstrom (1989)	1st UTI, birth to 6 y, temp 38.5°C	IVP, VCUG	32%	2%	3%
Marild (1989)	1st UTI, birth to 6 y, temp 38.5°C	IVP ± VCUG	26%	0	6.9%
Rickwood (1992)	1st/recurrent UTI, birth to 10 y	IVP/RI, US ± VCUG	24%	3%	15%
Riccabona (1991)	1st UTI, <1 y	US, VCUG	40%	—	—
Johnson (1985)	1st/recurrent UTI, 2 to 13 y	IVP, US, VCUG	16%	1.6%	1.6%
Messi (1989)	1st/recurrent UTI, birth to 15 y	IVP ± VCUG	18%	1.3%	1.7%

UTI, urinary tract infarction; RI, radionucleotide cortical imaging; IVP, intravenous pyelogram; US, ultrasound; VCUG, voiding cystourethrogram; RI/IVP, indicates that either RI or IVP was performed.

This review found no intervention studies. Most studies focused on the prevalence of urologic abnormalities, not on the effect that early detection and management of anomalies might have on outcomes. None of the studies found any direct evidence to support or reject the effectiveness of routine diagnostic imaging. The authors looked at the evidence for what they considered the three main questions relating to this issue:

What is the prevalence and severity of anomalies in children with UTIs? The table addresses this question. How long these outcomes had existed before the infection becoming clinically apparent is unknown. Whether children without UTIs also have these abnormalities is unknown.

What is the risk of adverse outcomes in children with the abnormalities described? Children followed for reflux can have progression or new scar formation during the years after initial diagnosis. This occurs primarily in children with additional UTIs during follow-up, however, or in children with a history of delay in diagnosis and treatment. These scars occurred primarily in children with four or more "pyelonephritic" infections. The risk for children of only one or two adequately managed UTIs may be minimal.

What is the effectiveness of early recognition and intervention? Two controlled trials showed that low-dose, long-term antimicrobial prophylaxis is efficacious in reducing UTI recurrences during a 1–2 year follow-up. Long-term prophylaxis also seems to reduce incidence of recurrent UTIs in children with vesicoureteral reflux compared with historical controls. Controlled trials of antimicrobial prophylaxis versus placebo in schoolgirls with asymptomatic bacteriuria failed to show an impact on renal scarring. The impact of long-term prophylaxis on renal scarring or outcomes such as hypertension in children has not been adequately tested. Surgical or endoscopic antireflux correction techniques reduce or eliminate reflux but have not been shown to reduce significantly renal scarring in moderately severe vesicoureteral reflux compared with antimicrobial prophylaxis in randomized controlled trials. Surgery may be more useful in severe cases, but no evidence is available.

Interpretation: Children with UTIs have a fairly high rate of urinary tract abnormalities at the time of diagnosis, but we do not know to what degree this is greater than in children without UTIs. The frequency of recurrence of UTIs and the severity of the UTIs (especially if the child is febrile) are associated with increased likelihood of renal scarring. A frequency of one or two mild UTIs has a low likelihood of scarring, whereas a frequency of three or four severe UTIs has a high likelihood of scarring.

Antimicrobial prophylaxis reduces the likelihood of infection in children with or without vesicoureteral reflux. Early diagnosis and treatment of infections probably decreases renal scarring. Corrective surgical or endoscopic procedures reduce or eliminate vesicoureteral reflux, but their effect on reducing renal scarring is no better than antimicrobial prophylaxis.

Most severe cases of anomalies and renal scarring are detected early, during infancy. Young age of first infection and infection in boys probably mean a higher likelihood of anomaly.

Bottom line: Children with severe (with fever) and recurrent UTIs probably need referral, especially if UTIs occur in early infancy or in boys. It is likely, however, that most UTIs in children can be treated with antimicrobial prophylaxis and early diagnosis and treatment of infections that do occur. Whether all children with a first UTI should be referred and imaged is unknown, but the evidence that does exist suggests a more selective approach is reasonable.

What did Dr. Sharpe do?

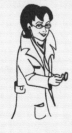

Dr. Sharpe decided that even if the culture is positive, she may treat Gemma and not refer at this point. Gemma's father was worried about the possibility of his daughter having invasive testing. There is little if any evidence to suggest that such testing would be of any benefit to Gemma. Dr. Sharpe thought she might get a noninvasive ultrasound done, treat Gemma for this infection, then wait and see. If the infection recurs, she will use antimicrobial prophylaxis and follow her with noninvasive techniques only. If the UTIs become severe and frequent, Dr. Sharpe will refer.

Reflection Exercise: How does this evidence apply to your practice? Would you apply this evidence to the management of appropriate patients in your practice? How will your practice change?

Citation: Colour vision screening: A critical appraisal of the literature. New Zealand Health Technology Assessment. The Clearinghouse for Health Outcomes and Health Technology Assessment, Department of Public Health and General Practice, Christchurch School of Medicine, Christchurch, NZ, October 1998, p. 23, 26.[19]

Studies: Six studies were identified that compared motor vehicle crash statistics between individuals with normal color vision and individuals with impaired color vision. Four of the studies did not find any differences between the groups. One study identified significantly more crashes in the colorblind group. The other study showed that protans (decreased sensitivity to red-sensitive cones) had more crashes than individuals with normal vision and deutans (decreased sensitivity to green-sensitive cones) under wet conditions.

In a study in Germany, 2058 motor vehicle crashes caused by male drivers were investigated for the effect impaired color vision had on the crash rates. A descriptive design was used. Motor vehicle crashes were caused by a color-deficient driver in 8.4% of the cases. Because this figure approximates the prevalence of impaired color vision among men, the authors concluded there was no evidence for an increased risk among this group. Protans had a higher proportion of their crashes resulting from rear-end collisions (43% versus 26% in normals, $p < 0.05$). This suggests the type of crash is different in the color-normal and color-deficient populations.

Interpretation: Color-deficient drivers do not seem to have more crashes than color-normal drivers, but the types of crashes may be different. Color-deficient drivers have more rear-end collisions. Perhaps the protans do not notice the red brake lights as easily as people with normal color vision.

What did Dr. Sharpe do?

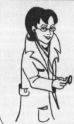

If Mr. Simms is colorblind, Dr. Sharpe will reassure him that he may not be more likely to have accidents, although he is more prone to rear-end collisions. She will tell him that she will have to report any color vision deficiency on the form from the licensing agency, and they will decide whether it affects his ability to get a license.

Reflection Exercise: How does this evidence apply to your practice? Would you apply this evidence to the management of appropriate patients in your practice? How will your practice change?

Simon Werston
(Gastroesophageal Reflux)

You had seen Simon Werston just once before, about a year ago, when he presented with mild heartburn. At that time, he described the heartburn as a retrosternal burning with sour regurgitation and belching that occurred after a large or spicy meal. It occurred about once or twice a week. He claimed to have had occasional heartburn for years, but it had increased over the previous year. There was nothing abnormal to find on abdominal examination at that time.

You told Mr. Werston that you thought the heartburn was esophageal reflux and explained what that was. You discussed smaller, more frequent meals and avoiding spicy foods and caffeine. You also advised he quit smoking, which he has not done.

Today, Mr. Werston says the frequency and severity of the heartburn have increased over the past 6 months. It now occurs daily and often awakens him at night. There is no association with exertion, and you do not think this is angina. He has gained 5 lb since his last visit. He has not been following your dietary advice.

You review your previous dietary advice, ask him again to consider quitting smoking, and tell him he should make an appointment specifically to discuss that issue. You explain the mechanism of esophageal reflux again and this time recommend he elevate the head of his bed to help prevent nighttime reflux. You prescribe ranitidine, 150 mg twice daily, and arrange a barium swallow and upper gastrointestinal series.

You know there are "alarm features" that need to be looked for in patients with gastroesophageal reflux disease (GERD)—dysphagia, weight loss, gastrointestinal bleeding, and failure to respond to an adequate trial of therapy. Mr. Werston does not have any of these features at this point. You have used cisapride in the past with other patients and often found it useful. You heard some reports, however, of potential problems with cisapride causing cardiac-related deaths. You wonder if there are other similar "prokinetic-type" agents available that are useful and that do not cause these side effects.

You ask Mr Werston to return in 2 weeks to let you know how the ranitidine is working and to discuss the results of his barium studies.

38 In a 34-year-old man with classic symptoms of GERD occurring daily, how well do barium studies diagnose the condition compared with endoscopy?

39 In a 34-year-old man with classic symptoms of GERD occurring daily, but who does not have any alarm features, what is the likelihood of a malignant lesion being present?

40 In a 34-year-old man with GERD, are there prokinetic agents available that are useful and that do not cause serious side effects?

Reflection Exercise:

What are your thoughts regarding these questions? Consider them in the context of your own practice. Consider what you might do before you read the evidence.

Answer to Questions 38, 39, and 40

Preamble

All three of these questions are addressed in this excellent evidence-based guideline.

Citation: Veldhuyzen van Zanten SJO, Flook N, Chiba N, et al. An evidence-based approach to the management of uninvestigated dyspepsia in the era of *Helicobacter pylori*. Can Med Assoc J 2000; 162(12 Suppl):S3–S24.[107]

Producers of the guideline: The guideline was produced by the Canadian Dyspepsia Working Group, which consists of 18 experts in dyspepsia, evidence-based medicine, and continuing medicine education. The group is a mixture of university-based and private practice family physicians, gastroenterologists, and pharmacists.

Databases searched: Medline 1966–1999. Searches were done on definition, classification, differential diagnosis, prevalence, natural history, prevalence of organic disease, and treatment of dyspepsia. The reference lists of key articles were searched.

Sources of evidence: High-quality reviews, systematic reviews, and meta-analyses were considered as sources of evidence. The original articles were retrieved and evaluated. Relevant studies were graded as to their strength of evidence.

Question 38: Endoscopy is superior to barium studies. The barium studies are neither sensitive nor specific. If the barium study is positive (suggests an ulcer), an endoscopy still needs to be done to assess whether it is a benign or malignant ulcer, especially if the ulcer is located in the stomach. If barium studies are negative, an endoscopy needs to be done because the barium study is not sensitive to rule out disease. Neither barium studies nor endoscopy needs to be done, however, unless there are *alarm* features—age >50 years, vomiting, bleeding, anemia, abdominal mass, unexplained weight loss, or dysphagia. If none of these features is present, the patient with dyspepsia can be treated without investigation. If treatment fails, investigation is needed even in patients without alarm features.

Question 39: The likelihood of a malignant lesion in a 34-year-old man with no alarm features is extremely low. In four prevalence studies assessing 5933 patients with dyspepsia, there were no cases of gastric or esophageal cancer in any patient <45 years old. In Canada, the probability of developing gastric cancer is 0.1% in men at age 50 years and approaching 0 at age 40 years. The guideline uses 50 years as the point when prompt investigation of new symptoms is justified.

Question 40: Cisapride is the only prokinetic agent that has been shown to be effective. Because cisapride has serious potential side effects and has been withdrawn from the market, GERD is best treated with proton-pump inhibitors or H_2 reuptake antagonists.

What did Dr. Sharpe do?

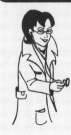

Dr. Sharpe had prescribed ranitidine, which was an appropriate treatment, although the efficacy of proton-pump inhibitors is greater. She also had arranged barium studies, but after reading the guideline, she wished she had not done that. She called Mr. Werston and suggested he not get the barium study done at this point but wait and see how he did with the medication. He agreed. If the ranitidine was not helpful, Dr. Sharpe would suggest an endoscopy.

Reflection Exercise: How does this evidence apply to your practice? Would you apply this evidence to the management of appropriate patients in your practice? How will your practice change?

INTERLUDE 3

On Friday evening at 8 PM at home, you receive a telephone call from Fitz. He wanted to let you know that although they had not yet located Leo Nash, his accomplice had been apprehended. It seemed that Joey Hynes was not the one with the brains in the duo and was a bit of a wimp. He had cracked easily when he was told they had evidence linking him and Leo to the two murders. He agreed to tell everything, if he could be guaranteed some sort of immunity. The police and Joey's lawyer had worked out an agreement, and Joey was going to give his statement officially the next morning in Toronto. Fitz was going to be there, and he had obtained approval for you to come along.

You drive to Toronto the next morning with Fitz. He was feeling better, he said, and hadn't had any more attacks. Fitz told you about Leo Nash and Joey Hynes. Leo was the dangerous one. Joey sort of went along for the ride. Fitz had heard they were gay, but he wasn't certain. They were both in their late 30s. Leo had broken into a house of an elderly couple many years ago. He had been caught by the old man, who had come downstairs when he heard a noise. Leo attacked the old man and beat him badly. Fortunately the wife, who had stayed upstairs, called the police, and they were there within minutes. The police apprehended Leo and got help for the old man. Leo had served time and was released 2 years ago.

Joey had spent a year in jail for petty theft. He had never been involved in any violence. He apparently met Leo just about a year ago. They struck up a relationship, and apparently Joey had helped Leo with a couple of "jobs."

At the police station in Toronto, Joey, his lawyer, one plainclothes police officer, and the crown attorney were in a separate room. You were watching what was happening on a television screen. There was a camera in the room, and everything was being taped. Viewing with you were Fitz, two other police officers, and to your surprise Nick Sampson and his lawyer. Nick had been brought in to see if he recognized Joey. If the police were satisfied with Joey's statement and it didn't implicate Nick in anyway, he then would be released.

The crown attorney, who obviously was well briefed on the known facts to date, led the questioning. In his own words, Joey's story went like this:

> Leo Nash asked me if I wanted to help him with a job that was going to pay big. He said it was worth $25,000, and he would give me $5000 if I helped him. I figured it meant blowing someone away for that kind of cash, but I went along with it anyway. I knew Leo would actually do it. I can't do it myself; Leo says I'm too much of a wimp. He told me the guy's name who was hiring him. He said it was a rich guy from Bedford, Pierre Savoy, and he wanted somebody named Amy Stephens quietly and simply gotten rid of and he didn't want the body ever to be found.

We met Savoy in his warehouse on Rodnam street. He asked Leo who I was, and Leo said I was his buddy who helped out with jobs. Savoy said the fee was the same even though there were two people, and Leo said yes he understood that. The deal was we were to get $5000 up front and the remaining $20,000 when the job was done. Savoy gave Leo the $5000 and told him the street address for Amy Stephens. The plan was for Leo to phone Amy and say that he was calling for Savoy. He was to tell her he would be along in Savoy's BMW to pick her up and bring her to Sak's Restaurant on Broad Street to meet with him. He said she would agree to come because of a financial deal they had and especially if he showed up in the BMW, which she would recognize. Savoy gave Leo a set of keys to his car. He said he would be away from June 8 to June 22 and that his car would be in the parking garage in the airport. Leo was supposed to get Savoy's car, and after calling Amy he was to go pick her up, do the deed without getting the car in a mess, dispose of the body, and then take the car back to the parking garage. The car would have to be back in the garage before 6 PM on Thursday, June 22, because that was when Savoy would be arriving back.

Leo didn't do anything that first week except get the car and drive it around. He liked the idea of driving around in a BMW—made him feel important. During that week, he asked around about Amy Stephens to see if anybody knew her. He discovered that she had been seeing Pierre Savoy and that now she was blackmailing him. Leo figured that was why he wanted her dead.

Anyway, Leo figured he had hit the jackpot and that we could get a lot more than $25,000. He would blackmail Savoy himself and soak him for everything he was worth. He would leave the body in the trunk of Savoy's car with a note. The note said to meet us at the corner of Yonge and Dundas to discuss the new deal. Leo was going to tell Savoy that we would get the body out of his car and dispose of it and keep this under wraps, but the price would be $50,000. The alternative would be for him to look after the body himself, but he could be sure the police would get an anonymous tip and they would find out about Amy's blackmail.

We waited for Savoy at Yonge and Dundas until 10:30 that night. He didn't show up. We didn't know what to do, so we did nothing. The next day Leo got a call from Savoy, and we met at the warehouse again. Savoy was angry. He asked what the hell the body was doing in Nick Sampson's car. Leo knew right away that we had put the body in the wrong car and Savoy hadn't got the note. Savoy said the deal was for the body to be disposed of, and now it was too late because the police already had the body. He said the price just dropped to $5000 and he had already paid that. They got into a shoving match, and Savoy caught his leg on a rusty nail and fell down. Leo put a gun to Savoy's head and said he wanted the full amount or the police would be fed information about Amy's blackmail, which would make Savoy a suspect. Savoy agreed but said he couldn't get back with the money for another 2 weeks because people were getting suspicious at home. Leo agreed with a warning that if he didn't show up he would come after him.

We read in the papers the next day about the body in Nick Sampson's car. We still don't know how that happened. But things sure got messed up. Then later we learned that the police had a note that had been left with the body. When Savoy met us again in the warehouse last weekend, we knew that he was a suspect as well as Nick Sampson. The story was getting out around town, and it was only a matter of time before the police knew. Leo figured that if Savoy was to end up killed, he would be dropped from the suspect list, and that might keep the police away from us. We had no connection with Nick Sampson, but we were connected with Savoy.

When Savoy arrived at the warehouse last Saturday, we were parked outside waiting. We all went inside; Savoy gave Leo the money in an envelope. Leo checked that it was all there and then without even a slight hesitation he pulled out a gun and shot him, twice in the head. He was dead before he hit the floor. I couldn't believe it. Now I was part of two murders.

I was getting worried. Then I heard that the police were looking for us. Leo heard about it too. He split. Before I could decide what to do the cops picked me up. I knew I had to come clean or I would be in bigger trouble. I didn't actually kill anybody. I was there when Leo strangled Amy Stephens, and I was there when Leo shot Savoy. But I didn't do it. I can't do that stuff.

The police officer asked Joey how they got Nick Sampson's car out without using the date-stamped ticket Sampson had obtained when he entered the parking garage.

Well, we drove to the airport in Leo's old car the day after Savoy and Sampson left town. We got one of those time-stamped tickets to get in and that was the one we used when we left in Sampson's car. Leo drove the car for almost 2 weeks around the city. But he always wore gloves. Smart, Leo is. Then when we took the car back with Amy's body in it, we got a time-stamped ticket going in and that was the one we used to get out in Leo's old car. Good trick, eh? I came up with that one!

The police officer asked how Leo and Joey got the car in and out without being seen and who the two women seen on the security camera were.

Leo and me dressed up as women. We figured we could fool the cops that way. Leo is an expert at cross-dressing. Since the security camera tapes only go back 1 week, we figured the tapes of us taking the car would be erased before anyone figured out you needed them.

Joey was asked how he and Leo managed to end up with Nick Sampson's car if they were supposed to get Pierre Savoy's car.

Leo is colorblind! When we went to pick up Savoy's car, there weren't many BMWs in the parking garage. Leo tried the keys in the first one he saw. I told him it was red and not green, but he tried the keys anyway and they worked. So I thought I must have heard Savoy wrong when I thought he said his car was green. I don't know why he gave us keys to Nick Sampson's car.

You turned to Fitz at this point and told him the story that Joanne had related to you about the keys she had left at Nancy's and how they subsequently worked in Pierre's car and not in Nick's. You both concluded that Pierre had given Leo Nash the wrong set of keys.

The interrogation went on a while longer, but it was mainly the same things over again. You were shown a picture of Leo Nash. Mug shots, face forward and in profile. You didn't recognize him. Nick didn't recognize him either, although he mentioned that Leo and Joey must have been on that corner, Yonge and Dundas, that same night that he was there waiting for whoever had left the note. They were waiting for someone they knew, though, and so paid no attention to him.

The police, after discussion with Nick and his lawyer, decided to let Nick go, as long as he agreed not to leave the area. They still needed to find Leo Nash.

Fitz wanted to stay in Toronto for a while longer, so you caught a ride back to Bedford with a happy Nick Sampson. Joanne and his parents would be much happier now. You thought of Nick's sister, Nancy Sampson-Savoy, and knew that next week was going to be difficult for her.

ACT IV

Jane Harris
(Osteoarthritis of the Hip)

Mrs. Harris is a widow. She has been complaining of left hip pain for many years. It is getting increasingly worse as the years go by. Recently the nonsteroidal anti-inflammatory drugs have not been working as well to relieve her pain, and she has taken to using a cane. She is in today because she is now having trouble getting upstairs to her bedroom and she is worried she will have to move out of her house, which she does not want to do.

You suggested hip replacement to Mrs. Harris in the past, but she did not want to pursue it, but that is exactly what she wants to discuss today. Her main concerns are success rate and complications. Apart from mild hypertension and osteoarthritis in other joints (right knee and hands), Mrs. Harris is healthy.

A question arising from this clinical encounter

41 In a 72-year-old woman who needs a total hip replacement owing to osteoarthritis, what are the success rate and complications rate?

Reflection Exercise:

What are your thoughts regarding this question? Consider this question in the context of your own practice. Consider what you might do before you read the evidence.

Answer to Question 41

Preamble

We review two articles on outcomes from total hip replacements. The first one looks at "hard" outcomes, such as mortality, infection rates, and revision rates. The second one looks at quality of life.

Citation: Kreder HJ, Williams JIW, Jaglal S, et al. Are complication rates for elective primary total hip arthroplasty in Ontario related to surgeon and Hospital volumes? Can J Surg 1998; 41:431–437.[57]

Study design: Retrospective population cohort study.

Population: Patients (3645) who had undergone elective total hip replacement in Ontario during 1992 as recorded in the Canadian Institute for Health Information database. The average age was 67 years, and 42% of patients were men.

Outcomes assessed: In-hospital complications, 1- and 3-year revision rates, 1- and 3-year infection rates, length of hospital stay, and 3-month and 1-year death rates.

The Evidence

Complications and Other Outcomes	Number and Percent out of 3645
Serious complication during initial procedure	319 (8.8%)
Died during initial hospitalization	13 (0.4%)
Discharged home (approx)	1531 (42%)
Died within 3 months of procedure	26 (0.7%)
Died within 1 year of procedure	61 (1.7%)
Readmitted within 1 year for infection in hip joint prosthesis infection	35 (1%)
Readmitted within 3 years for infection in hip joint prosthesis infection	70 (1.9%)
Readmitted within 1 year for a revision of the procedure	44 (1.2%)
Readmitted within 3 years for a revision of the procedure	80 (2.2%)

Patient comorbidity was significantly associated with 1-year mortality.

Interpretation: Complication rates were low. Nearly 60% of patients were not discharged home, however, meaning they died in the hospital (0.4%), were discharged to a nursing home, or were transferred to another institution, such as a rehabilitation hospital. The success rate as measured by patients not needing a revision within 3 years was high (97.8%).

Bottom line: Although there are definite risks, total hip replacement surgery is successful in most patients.

Citation: Knutsson S, Engberg IB. An evaluation of patients' quality of life before, 6 weeks, and 6 months after total hip replacement surgery. J Adv Nurs 1999; 30:1349–1359.[56]

Study design: Prospective assessment of quality of life before and after hip surgery. The Sickness Impact Profile (SIP) was the instrument used.

Study population: Patients (51) having hip surgery during the period September–November 1993 in three orthopedic wards of a large hospital in western Sweden. Of the 51 patients completing the questionnaire before surgery, 47 completed it 6 weeks postoperatively, and 40 completed it 6 months postoperatively.

The Evidence

Non-SIP Factors	Before Surgery	6 Weeks Postop.	6 Months Postop.
Pain-free	0%	35 (75%)	21 (52%)
Walk without ambulation support (e.g., cane or walker)	—	20 (43%)	31 (78%)

SIP Factor	Quality of Life at 6 Weeks Compared with Preop.	Quality of Life at 6 Months Compared with Preop.
Sleep/rest	Improved	Further improvement
Emotional behavior	Improved	Further improvement
Body/care/movement	Unchanged	Improved
Home management	Worse	Improved
Mobility	Worse	Improved
Social interaction	Slightly improved	Further slight improvement
Ambulation	Slightly worse	Improved
Alertness behavior	Very slightly improved	Very slightly worse
Communication	Very slightly worse	Unchanged
Work	Worse	Much better
Recreation/pastime	Improved	Further improvement
Eating	Slightly worse	Unchanged
Overall physical index	Worse	Better
Overall psychosocial index	Improved	Further improvement
Total SIP index	Worse	Improved

Interpretation: On functional and quality-of-life scores, patients generally improved with surgery, but this was more apparent at 6 months than at 6 weeks. At 6 weeks, the patients still were recovering, and certain factors were worse.

Bottom line: Hip replacement leads to improvement in function and quality of life by 6 months postoperatively.

What did Dr. Sharpe do?

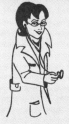

Mrs. Harris's questions were mainly about complications and success rate. Dr. Sharpe told Mrs. Harris that although significant complications could occur in about 8.8% of patients while in the hospital, the death rate was very low in the hospital and during the first year postoperatively. Dr. Sharpe also told her that 1–2% of patients were readmitted to the hospital within 3 years for reoperation or because of infection in the prosthesis. She told Mrs. Harris that her overall quality of life was likely to be improved significantly by 6 months postoperatively and that pain was likely to be improved sooner than that.

Reflection Exercise: How does this evidence apply to your practice? Would you apply this evidence to the management of appropriate patients in your practice? How will your practice change?

Mary Collier
(Chronic Obstructive Pulmonary Disease)

Mary Collier has been a smoker all her life. For 10 years, she has been getting more short of breath. She is on maximum doses of ipratropium bromide (Atrovent) and albuterol (Ventolin). She continues to be limited by her breathing capacity. You wonder about theophyllines and steroids. You know steroids are used in asthma but not in chronic obstructive pulmonary disease (COPD) generally. You also recall that theophyllines used to be used for COPD, and you wonder what the latest is on their use in this condition.

A question arising from this clinical encounter

42 In a 52-year-old woman with COPD on maximum doses of ipratropium bromide and albuterol, would oral or inhaled steroids or oral theophylline decrease shortness of breath and increase functional capacity?

Reflection Exercise:

What are your thoughts regarding this question? Consider this question in the context of your own practice. Consider what you might do before you read the evidence.

Answer to Question 42

Citation: Barr RG, Rowe BH, Camargo CA. Methylxanthines for exacerbations of chronic obstructive pulmonary disease. Cochrane Review. In: The Cochrane Library, Issue 1. Oxford: Update Software; 2001.[9]

Study design: Systematic review with meta-analysis.

Data sources: MEDLINE, EMBASE, CINAHL, CENTRAL, and hand searching of 20 respiratory journals and bibliographies from included studies and known reviews.

Number of studies: 4

Number of patients: 172

Time frame: 1996–2001

Article selection criteria: Randomized controlled trials only were looked at, in which patients presented with acute exacerbations of COPD and were treated with either methylxanthine (oral or intravenous) or placebo (with or without usual care). Outcomes had to be pulmonary function or admission results. Two reviewers independently selected potentially relevant articles.

Data extraction: Data were extracted independently by two reviewers. Missing data were obtained from authors or calculated from other data in the article.

Article appraisal process: Quality was assessed independently by two reviewers.

Statistical heterogeneity tests? Yes ($p < 0.01$).

Publication bias testing? No.

The Evidence: Dichotomous Outcomes

Outcome	EER	CER	Peto Odds Ratio	ARR	NNTh
Hospital admissions	2 of 23 (8.7%)	4 of 16 (25%)	0.29 (0.05–1.80)	NA	NA
Emergency department returns within 1 week	7 of 90 (7.7%)	6 of 95 (6.3%)	1.55 (0.48–4.99)	NA	NA
Proportion of patients with improvement in symptom score	68 of 78 (87.2%)	56 of 75 (74.6%)	2.38 (1.01–5.60)	12.6%	8
Nausea/vomiting	12 of 93 (12.9%)	2 of 88 (22.7%)	5.29 (1.33–21.0)	9.8%	10

EER, experimental event rate; CER, control event rate; ARR, absolute risk reduction; NNTh, number needed to treat to harm 1 person; NA, not applicable as there is no significant difference.

The Evidence: Continuous Outcomes

Outcome	Mean Difference in FEV_1 between the Groups	95% Confidence Interval of This Mean Difference	P Value
FEV_1 at 2 h	−8.21	−85–68	>0.05 (NS)

FEV_1, forced expiratory volume in 1 second; NS, not significant.

Interpretation: There seems to be no substantial effect of methylxanthines in the situation of acute exacerbation of COPD except to increase nausea. There was a slight increase in improvement in symptom scores. Part of the problem with this review is the lack of power created by so few studies. Only one study looked at hospital admission rate; it showed a 16% reduction in admission rates with methylxanthines, which seems to be clinically significant. Because of the small sample size, this rate did not achieve statistical significance.

Bottom line: Methylxanthines (oral or intravenous) have little, if any, effect on the outcome of acute exacerbations of COPD.

Citation: Wood-Baker R, Walters EH, Gibson P. Corticosteroids for acute exacerbations of chronic obstructive pulmonary disease. Cochrane Review. In: The Cochrane Library, Issue 1. Oxford: Update Software; 2001.[111]

Study design: Systematic review with meta-analysis.

Data sources: Cochrane Airways group COPD randomized controlled trial registry, search of bibliographies of articles, and contacted authors.

Number of studies: 7

Number of patients: 172

Time frame: 1996–2001

Article selection criteria: Randomized controlled trials only were looked at, in which patients presented with acute exacerbations of COPD and were treated with either corticosteroid (oral or intravenous) or placebo (with or without usual care).

Data extraction: Data were extracted by one of the reviewers and sent to authors for verification.

Statistical heterogeneity tests? Yes ($p < 0.01$).

The Evidence: Dichotomous Outcomes

Outcome	EER	CER	Peto Odds Ratio	ARR	NNTh
Treatment failure	8 of 67 (11.9%)	15 of 56 (26.7%)	0.40 (1.16–1.0)	14.8%	7
Mortality	5 of 165 (3.0%)	6 of 143 (4.2%)	0.73 (0.22–2.49)	NA	NA

EER, experimental event rate; CER, control event rate; ARR, absolute risk reduction; NNTh, number needed to treat to harm 1 person; NA, not applicable as there is no significant difference.

The Evidence: Continuous Outcomes

Outcome	Mean Difference between the Groups	95% Confidence Interval of This Mean Difference	P Value
Early FEV$_1$ (L)	−0.08	−0.18–0.02	>0.05 (NS)
Late FEV$_1$ (L)	−0.03	−0.21–0.15	>0.05 (NS)
Duration of hospitalization (days)	0.89	−2.87–4.65	>0.05 (NS)

FEV$_1$, forced expiratory volume in 1 second; NS, not significant.

Interpretation: Corticosteroids seem to have no significant effect on acute exacerbations of COPD.

Bottom line: Corticosteroids seem to have no significant effect on acute exacerbations of COPD.

What did Dr. Sharpe do?

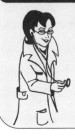

Although these reviews addressed acute exacerbations of COPD rather than poorly controlled COPD, Dr. Sharpe decided to apply the results to her patient. She did not start Mrs. Collier on theophylline or corticosteroids.

Reflection Exercise: How does this evidence apply to your practice? Would you apply this evidence to the management of appropriate patients in your practice? How will your practice change?

Leonard's Surprise
(Colorblindness)

It was the last patient of the day and of the week. Only you and Jonathon Simple had a clinic that afternoon, and Jon had finished up by 4 PM and gone home. The other two physicians were either taking their CME afternoon or getting an early start to what looked to be a great weekend.

Leonard Nelson was your last patient. He was scheduled for 4:30 PM, but you were a bit behind, and it was 5:15 PM. Jenny, the nurse, had told the receptionist to go home, and she would look after closing up when the last patient was finished.

As was the usual practice, Jenny had called Mr. Nelson into the examining room, determined the reason for the visit, checked vitals signs, and made a note on the chart. She passed you the chart in the hallway as you headed for the examining room. Jenny's note just said "colorblind, needs check for work, Ishihara charts in the room."

You walked into the room, sat down at your desk, and knew immediately that something was terribly wrong!

Some questions arising from this clinical encounter

43 What is the sensitivity and specificity of the Ishihara charts for detecting colorblindness?

Reflection Exercise:

What are your thoughts regarding this question? Consider this question in the context of your own practice. Consider what you might do before you read the evidence.

Answer to Question 43

Citation: Colour vision screening: A critical appraisal of the literature. New Zealand Health Technology Assessment. p. 23, 26.[19]

This review reported on four studies that looked at the sensitivity and specificity of the Ishihara tests.

The Evidence

Study	Sensitivity (%)	Specificity (%)
Pease and Allen	96	100
Dain et al (1997)	98	100
Hill et al (1982)	79	85
Ganlkey and Lian (1997)	100	98

Interpretation: The Ishihara charts can assess color vision accurately.

What did Dr. Sharpe do?

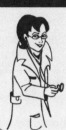

Not much! She didn't have the opportunity to test the patient's vision.

Reflection Exercise: How does this evidence apply to your practice? Would you apply this evidence to the management of appropriate patients in your practice? How will your practice change?

AFTERLUDE

It became known as the Bedford murder even though there were two murders and they happened in Toronto. But the final episode in the case was played out in Bedford and involved a death, although not technically a murder.

As the plane circled for landing, you remembered when you first arrived in Bedford. The streets were still laid out below in that perfect gridlike pattern. Houses in neat little rows with manicured lawns with the blue of swimming pools dotted here and there in a random pattern. The land was flat for miles around with a mixture of farmland and wooded areas. The slight bump of the landing brought you out of your reverie.

It had been 2 weeks since Leonard Nelson arrived at the clinic. The next day you had gone home to your parents to recover. You felt much better now, but you needed to talk to someone who understood the context of what had happened. After taking a taxi to your house, you called Jonathon. He invited you over for a beer and maybe to order out some food. Jonathon was a great friend, always ready to listen and help if he could.

As that mellow feeling from the lager began to encompass you, you told Jonathon the whole story.

As soon as you sat down at the desk in the examining room and looked at Leonard Nelson, you knew who he was—not Leonard Nelson at all, but Leo Nash. The police had been looking for him for several weeks. You had seen his mug shots in the police station in Toronto, and now he was here setting across from you. He obviously saw your look of recognition; he said, "Hello, bitch, I hear you're the one who turned me in."

You had never felt fear like that before. This man had killed two people within the past month, and now he was sitting in front of you with revenge on his mind. You felt panic rising inside you, but you controlled it. You said, "I'm sorry, what do you mean?"

But as you were saying it, you were remembering that you had only been lukewarm about the idea of installing those push-button alarms under the desks in each room. It had been costly, and you had wondered whether it was worth it. Now it might save your life. You reached in slowly and pressed the button. He didn't seem to notice. What he did do was slowly pull a gun from his inside pocket. "You know what I mean, and it's payback time."

Just as he raised the gun toward you, Jenny rushed through the door. She had seen the light, had pushed the button that called the police, then headed straight for the examining room. Jenny's entrance caused him to turn quickly toward the door. As he did, you grabbed the small Styrofoam cup half full of liquid nitrogen that was sitting on the desk. The last patient had been in for a wart treatment. You grabbed the cup as his attention was distracted and threw the liquid nitrogen in his face.

Both his hands went to his face, and you jumped toward him. He screamed and gave you a shove and pulled the trigger. There was a scream from Jenny as the bullet hit her upper left arm and shattered the bone. You lunged back at him and the gun flew from his hand. He still couldn't see very well, but well enough to chase you as you ran from the room. Jenny, still in pain and weak, stretched out her leg and tripped him as he ran after you. He sprawled out into the hallway. He got up screaming and cursing and went back into the room to finish Jenny off with his bare hands. His hands were around her neck when you came back into the room and hit him over the head with the only weapon you could find, a pitcher that was still holding a bouquet of flowers. The pitcher shattered. Chrysanthemums, daisies, and baby's breath sprinkled everywhere as Leo Nash slumped over holding his head. There was a lot of blood, from Jenny's arm and Leo Nash's head. You were short of breath and high on adrenaline as you watched him stumble to the floor face down. Just as you relaxed, you saw him, as if in slow motion, roll over and point the gun straight at you. His last words were, "'Bye, bitch," just as Fitz shot him from the doorway, right through the middle of his forehead.

The police called the ambulance. You and Jenny were taken to the hospital. Jenny required transfer to Kingston for some major bone reconstruction surgery on her arm. You were fine, just a bit shaken. But you took the advice of the other doctors and your friends who encouraged you to take some time off.

It was the right thing to do. You had spent lots of time resting, chatting with your parents, going for long walks in the park and around the neighborhood you had played in as a child. You felt good now. Ready to get back to work. You thought you could talk about the incident without emotion now, and this little test run on Jonathon had proved that to be correct. You also realized how much you liked Bedford despite the incident that had almost cost you your life. You liked the people, the work, and your friends. You thought you might stay a while.

APPENDIX 1

Understanding the Evidence Tables

We have used several types of tables to present the evidence in this book. The type of table is dictated by the type of study. *Randomized controlled trials* (RCTs) and *systematic reviews with meta-analysis* (SR/M) have different types of tables, as do articles that study diagnostic tests.

Randomized Controlled Trials: The following table is the most common type, presenting the evidence from an RCT. It presents dichotomous outcomes (i.e., outcomes that are measured as yes or no, present or not present): for instance, myocardial infarction—it either happened or it didn't. This type of table presents the number of times the outcome happened in the experimental group and the number of times it happened in the control group. Although RCTs can produce outcomes that are continuous (e.g., forced vital capacity or forced expiratory volume in 1 second) and have means and standard deviations, all the RCTs in this book have dichotomous outcomes. The SR/M in this book have dichotomous and continuous outcomes, and they are described later.

Randomized Controlled Trial Dichotomous Outcomes

Outcome	EER (Intervention)	CER (Conventional)	Relative Risk	ARR	NNTb
Any diabetes-related end point	963 of 2729 (35.3%)	438 of 1138 (38.5%)	0.91 (0.81–1.0)	NA	NA
Diabetes-related deaths	285 of 2729 (10.4%)	129 of 1138 (11.3%)	0.92 (0.75–1.12)	NA	NA
All-cause mortality	489 of 2729 (17.8%)	213 of 1138 (18.7%)	0.95 (0.72–1.10)	NA	NA
Myocardial infarction	387 of 2729 (14.2%)	186 of 1138 (16.3%)	0.87 (0.74–1.03)	NA	NA
Stroke	148 of 2729 (5.4%)	55 of 1138 (4.8%)	0.88 (0.84–1.49)	NA	NA
Amputation or death from PVD	29 of 2729 (1%)	18 of 1138 (1.6%)	0.62 (0.33–1.20)	NA	NA
Microvascular	225 of 2729 (8.2%)	121 of 1138 (10.6%)	0.77 (0.62–0.97)	2.4%	42

EER, experimental event rate; CER, control event rate; ARR, absolute risk reduction; NNTb, number needed to treat to benefit 1 person; NA, not applicable as there is no significant difference; PVD, peripheral vascular disease.

The *experimental event rate (EER)* is the proportion or percentage of times the outcome occurred in the experimental group. Using the example of myocardial infarction in the table, 387 people out of the 2729 people in the experimental group had a myocardial infarction during the course of the study. This means 387/2729 or 14.2% of people in that group had a myocardial infarction.

The *control event rate (CER)* is the proportion or percentage of times the outcome occurred in the control group. Again using the example of myocardial infarction in the table, 186 people out of the 1138 people in the control group had a myocardial infarction during the course of the study. This means 186/1138 or 16.3% of people in that group had a myocardial infarction.

The *relative risk (RR)* is the EER/CER, which in the example is 14.2/16.3 or 0.142/0.163 = 0.87. This means that a patient is only 87% as likely to have a myocardial infarction if they receive the experimental treatment compared with people who receive the control treatment; this is an improvement with treatment. But is it a significant improvement? For that we look at the confidence interval.

The *95% confidence interval* is given in parentheses after the RR. If this confidence interval includes 1 (i.e., if the upper limit is ≥1), the effect (the improvement) is not significant. For myocardial infarction, the confidence interval is 0.74 to 1.03. It includes 1 and is not significant. When the confidence interval includes 1 and the improvement is not significant, we do not give absolute risk reduction (ARR) or number-needed-to-treat (NNT) because they have no meaning. There is no risk reduction.

The *absolute risk reduction (ARR)* is the absolute amount the risk of the outcome was decreased. It is calculated by CER − EER. For the outcome "Microvascular" in the table, the ARR is 10.6 − 8.2 = 2.4%. So the likelihood of a person having a microvascular complication is 2.4% less if a person receives the experimental treatment compared with a person who receives the control treatment.

The *number-needed-to-treat (NNT)* is the number of people who would have to receive the experimental treatment as opposed to the control treatment for one person not to have the outcome (e.g., for one person not to have a microvascular complication). It is calculated by 1/ARR (i.e., 1/0.024 or 100/2.4 = 42).

Systematic Reviews with Meta-Analysis: The following table is the most common type of table presenting the evidence from an SR/M. It presents dichotomous outcomes (i.e., outcomes that are measured as yes or no, present or not present): for instance, uterine rupture—it either happened or it didn't. This type of table presents the number of times the outcome happened in the experimental groups and the number of times it happened in the control groups of the studies in the review. In contrast to the table presenting dichotomous outcomes from a single RCT, which uses RR to compare the relative effectiveness of the experimental treatment with the control treatment, in SR/M, an odds ratio (OR) is used. A special type of OR is used in SR/M called the *Peto odds ratio.*

Systematic Review with Meta-Analysis Dichotomous Outcomes

Outcome	EER (Trial of Labor)	CER (Elective Repeat Section)	Peto Odds Ratio	ARR	NNTh
Uterine rupture	77 of 17,613 (0.4%)	22 of 11,433 (0.2%)	2.1 (1.45–3.05)	0.2%	500
Maternal mortality	3 of 27,504 (0.01%)	0 of 11,433 (0)	1.52 (0.36–6.38)	NA	NA
5-minute APGAR score < 7	41 of 1830 (2%)	14 of 1483 (0.9%)	2.24 (1.29–3.88)	1.1%	91

EER, experimental event rate; CER, control event rate; ARR, absolute risk reduction; NNTh, number needed to treat to harm 1 person; NA, not applicable as there is no significant difference.

The *EER* is the proportion or percentage of times the outcome occurred in the experimental group (trial of labor group) in the studies in the review. Using the example of uterine rupture in the table, 77 people out of the 17,613 people in the trial of labor group had a uterine rupture during the course of the study. This means 77/17,613 or 0.4% of people in that group had a uterine rupture.

The *CER* is the proportion or percentage of times the outcome occurred in the control (elective repeat [cesarean] section) group. Again using the example of uterine rupture in the table, 22 people out of the 11,433 people in the elective repeat section group had a uterine rupture during the course of the study. This means 22/11,433 or 0.2% of people in that group had a uterine rupture.

The *Peto odds ratio (OR)* can be understood in a similar manner as the RR. In this case, the event occurs more often in the experimental group, however, so the OR is greater than 1—it is 2.1. The outcome, uterine rupture, occurs 2.1 times more often in the experimental group (trial of labor) than in the control group (elective repeat section). So, is this a significant increase in this adverse outcome? For that we look at the confidence interval.

The *95% confidence interval* is given in parentheses after the Peto OR. If this confidence interval includes 1 (i.e., if the lower limit is ≤1), the effect (the increase) is not significant. For uterine rupture, the confidence interval is 1.45 to 3.05. It does not include 1 and is statistically significant. But is it clinically significant? For that we need absolute risk increase (ARI) and NNT.

The *absolute risk increase (ARI)* is the absolute amount the risk of the outcome was increased. It is calculated by CER − EER; the negative sign is ignored, so it is the absolute value of CER − EER. For the outcome uterine rupture in the table, the ARI is 0.2% − 0.4% = − 0.2% = 0.2%. So the likelihood of a person having a uterine rupture complication is 0.2% more if a person has a trial of labor compared with a person who has an elective repeat section.

The *NNT* is the number of people who would have to have a trial of labor as opposed to having an elective repeat section for one person to have a uterine rupture. It is calculated by 1/ARR (i.e., 1/0.002 or 100/0.2 = 500).

Sometimes an SR/M reports continuous outcomes. This is often presented as the mean differences between the outcomes in the experimental group and the control group. In the following table, the number of minutes it took people to go to sleep after taking a benzodiazepine was the outcome of interest. It took people on average 4.2 fewer minutes to fall asleep if they took a benzodiazepine compared with people who took a placebo. The confidence interval was −0.7 minutes to +9.2 minutes. When you are looking at differences, 0 is the equivalency point rather than 1. If the confidence interval includes 0, the difference is not statistically significant.

Systematic Review with Meta-Analysis Continuous Outcomes

Outcome	Mean Difference (Treatment − Placebo) with 95% Confidence Intervals	P Value
Sleep latency (time it took to get to sleep) (min)	−4.2 (−0.7–9.2)	NS
Total sleep duration (min)	61.8 (37.4–86.2)	<0.05

NS, not significant.

Studies of Diagnostic Tests: Studies looking at diagnostic tests compare them with a gold standard and provide sensitivity, specificity, and likelihood ratios: for instance, the study of the Ottawa ankle rules in the following table.

Outcome of Ankle Injuries

	Fracture on X-Ray	No Fracture on X-Ray	Total
Ankle rules positive for fracture a b	48	171	219
Ankle rules negative for fracture c d	1	137	138
Total	49	308	357

Sensitivity = a/a+c = 98%; specificity = d/b+d = 44%; positive predictive value = a/a+b = 22%; negative predictive value = d/c+d = 99%; positive likelihood ratio = sensitivity/1 − specificity = 176; negative likelihood ratio = 1 − sensitivity/specificity = 0.05.

Glossary of Terms in Evidence-Based Medicine

Not all of the following terms are used in this book.

Absolute risk reduction (ARR): The difference in the event rate between control group (CER) and treated group (EER): ARR = CER − EER. It tells us the absolute percent by which an intervention or exposure decreases the likelihood of the outcome. If the outcome being studied is considered bad or unwanted, such as a myocardial infarction, the ARR is used to calculate an NNTb (number needed to treat to benefit one person). If the outcome being studied is considered good or desired, such as a control of pain, the ARR is used to calculate an NNTh (number needed to treat to harm one person).

Absolute risk increase (ARI) is calculated in the same way as ARR but is used when the ARR is negative; the absolute value of the ARR is used and is called the ARI. The intervention increases the rate of the outcome rather than decreasing it. If the outcome being studied is considered bad or unwanted, such as a myocardial infarction, the ARI is used to calculate an NNTh. If the outcome being studied is considered good or desired, such as a control of pain, the ARI is used to calculate an NNTb.

Bias: Any tendency to influence the results of a trial (or their interpretation) other than the experimental intervention.

Blinding: A technique used in research to eliminate bias by hiding the intervention from the patient, clinician, or other researchers who are interpreting results.

Blobbogram: A diagrammatic representation of the results of individual trials in a systematic review.

Case-control: A study that involves identifying patients who have the outcome of interest (cases) and control patients without the same outcome and looking back to see if they had the exposure of interest.

Case-series: A report on a series of patients with an outcome of interest. No control group is involved.

Clinical practice guideline: A systematically developed statement designed to assist the practitioner and patient in making decisions about appropriate health care for specific clinical circumstances.

Cochrane Collaboration: A worldwide association of groups that create and maintain systematic reviews of the literature for a specific topic area.

Cohort study: Involves identifying two groups (cohorts) of patients, one that did receive the exposure of interest and one that did not, and following these cohorts forward for the outcome of interest.

Confidence interval (CI): The range around a study's result within which we would expect the true value to lie. CIs account for the sampling error between the study population and the wider population the study is supposed to represent.

Confounding variable: A variable that is not the one you are interested in but that may affect the results of a study.

Control event rate: See **Event rate.**

Cost-benefit analysis: Converts effects into the same monetary terms as the costs and compares them.

Cost-effectiveness analysis: Converts effects into health terms and describes the costs for some additional health gain (e.g., cost per additional myocardial infarction prevented).

Cost-utility analysis: Converts effects into personal preferences (or utilities) and describes how much it costs for some additional quality gain (e.g., cost per additional quality-adjusted life-year).

Critically appraised topic: A short summary of an article from the literature, created to answer a specific clinical question.

Crossover study design: The administration of two or more experimental therapies one after the other in a specified or random order to the same group of patients.

Cross-sectional study: The observation of a defined population at a single point in time or time interval. Exposure and outcome are determined simultaneously.

Decision analysis: The application of explicit, quantitative methods to analyze decisions under conditions of uncertainty.

Ecologic survey: Based on aggregated data for some population as it exists at some point or points in time; to investigate the relationship of an exposure to a known or presumed risk factor for a specified outcome.

Event rate: The proportion of patients in a group in whom the event is observed. If out of 100 patients, the event is observed in 27, the event rate is 0.27. **Control event rate (CER)** and **experimental event rate (EER)** are used to refer to this in control and experimental groups of patients.

Evidence-based health care: Extends the application of the principles of **evidence-based medicine** to all professions associated with health care, including purchasing and management.

Evidence-based medicine (EBM): The conscientious, explicit, and judicious use of current best evidence in making decisions about the care of individual patients. The practice of EBM means integrating individual clinical expertise with the best available external clinical evidence from systematic research.

Experimental event rate: See **Event rate.**

f: An estimate of the chance of an event for a patient, expressed as a decimal fraction of the control group's risk (event rate).

Funnel plot: A method of graphing the results of trials in a systematic review to show if the results have been affected by publication bias.

Gold standard: see **Reference standard.**

Heterogeneity: In systematic reviews, the amount of incompatibility between trials included in the review, whether clinical (i.e., the studies are clinically different) or statistical (i.e., the results are different from one another).

Intention-to-treat: A type of study in which patients are analyzed in the groups to which they were originally assigned, even though they may have switched treatment arms during the study for clinical reasons.

Likelihood ratio: The likelihood that a given test result would be expected in a patient with the target disorder compared with the likelihood that the same result would be expected in a patient without that disorder.

MeSH (Medical Subject Headings): A thesaurus of medical terms used by many databases and libraries to index and classify medical information.

Meta-analysis: An overview that uses quantitative methods to summarize the results.

N-of-1 trials: The patient undergoes pairs of treatment periods organized so that one period involves the use of the experimental treatment and one period involves the use of an alternate or placebo therapy. The patients and physician are blinded, if possible, and outcomes are monitored. Treatment periods are replicated until the clinician and patient are convinced that the treatments are definitely different or definitely not different.

Negative predictive value (−PV): The proportion of people with a negative test result who are free of disease.

Number needed to treat (NNT): The number of patients who need to be treated to prevent one bad outcome. It is the inverse of ARR: NNT = 1/ARR.

Odds: A ratio of nonevents to events. If the event rate for a disease is 0.1 (10%), its nonevent rate is 0.9, and its odds are 9:1. This is not the same expression as the inverse of event rate.

Odds ratio (OR): Describes the odds of an experimental patient suffering an adverse event relative to a control patient.

Overview: A summary of medical literature in a particular area.

P value: The probability that a particular result would have happened by chance.

Patient expected event rate (PEER): An estimate of the risk of an outcome for a patient.

Placebo: An inactive version of the active treatment that is administered to patients so that they do not know whether or not they are receiving the experimental treatment.

Positive predictive value (+PV): The proportion of people with a positive test result who have disease.

Prevalence: The baseline risk of a disorder in the population of interest.

Pretest probability: The probability that a patient has the disorder of interest before administering a test.

Posttest probability: The probability that a patient has the disorder of interest after the test result is known.

Publication bias: A bias in a systematic review caused by incompleteness of the search, such as omitting non–English language sources or unpublished trials (inconclusive trials are less likely to be published than conclusive ones, but are not necessarily less valid).

Randomized controlled clinical trial (RCT): A group of patients is randomized into an experimental group and a control group. These groups are followed up for the variables and outcomes of interest.

Reference standard: A diagnostic test used in trials to confirm presence or absence of the target disorder.

Relative risk reduction (RRR): The percent reduction in events in the treated group EER compared with the CER: RRR = (CER − EER) / CER · 100.

Risk: The probability that an event will occur for a particular patient or group of patients. Risk can be expressed as a decimal fraction or percentage (0.25 = 25%).

Risk ratio (RR): The ratio of risk in the treated group (EER) to the risk in the control group (CER): RR = EER/CER. RR is used in randomized trials and cohort studies.

Sensitivity: The proportion of people with disease who have a positive test.

SnNout: When a sign or test has a high sensitivity, a negative result rules out the diagnosis (e.g., the sensitivity of a history of ankle swelling for diagnosing ascites is 92%; if a person does not have a history of ankle swelling, it is highly unlikely that the person has ascites).

Specificity: The proportion of people free of a disease who have a negative test.

Spectrum bias: A bias caused by a study population whose disease profile does not reflect those of the intended population (e.g., if they have more severe forms of the disorder).

SpPin: When a sign or test has a high specificity, a positive result rules in the diagnosis (e.g., the specificity of fluid wave for diagnosing ascites is 92%; if a person has a fluid wave, it is highly likely that the person has ascites).

Systematic review (SR): An article in which the authors have systematically searched for, appraised, and summarized all of the medical literature for a specific topic.

References and Suggested Readings

1. Alaster JJ, Wood MD. Drug therapy. N Engl J Med 1993; 328:1398–1405.
2. American Diabetes Association. Standards of medical care for patients with diabetes mellitus. Diabetes Care 1998; 21(Suppl 1):S23–S31.
3. Assendelft WJ, Hay EM, Adshead R, Bouter LM. Corticosteroid injections for lateral epicondylitis: A systematic review. Br J Gen Pract 1996; 46:209–216.
4. Assman G, Cullen P, Schulte H. The Munster Heart Study (PROCAM): Results of follow-up at 8 years. Eur Heart J 1998; 19(Suppl A):A2–A11.
5. Auleley GR, Kerboull L, Durieux P, et al. Validation of the Ottawa Ankle Rules in France: A study in the surgical emergency department of teaching hospital. Ann Emerg Med 1998; 32:15–18.
6. Azais-Braesco V, Pascal G. Vitamin A in pregnancy: Requirements and safety limits. Am J Clin Nutr 2000; 71(Suppl):1325S–1333S.
7. Badenoch D, Sackett D, Strauss S, et al. CatMaker. Oxford: Centre for Evidence Based Medicine; Copyright 2000. Available at http://cebm.jr2.ox.ac.uk.
8. Baker B, Paquette M, Szalai JP, et al. The influence of marital adjustment on 3-year left ventricular mass and ambulatory blood pressure in mild hypertension. Arch Intern Med 2000; 160:3453–3458.
9. Barr RG, Rowe BH, Camargo CA. Methylxanthines for exacerbations of chronic obstructive pulmonary disease. Cochrane Review. In: The Cochrane Library, Issue 1. Oxford: Update Software; 2001.
10. Barratt A, Irwig L, Glasziou P, et al. Users' guides to medical literature: XVII. How to use guidelines and recommendations about screening. JAMA 1999; 281:2029.
11. Brocklehurst P, Hannah M, McDonald H: Interventions for treating bacterial vaginosis in pregnancy. Cochrane review. In: The Cochrane Library, Issue 4. Oxford: Update Software; 2000.
12. Bucher HC, Guyatt GH, Cook DJ, et al. Users' guides to the medical literature: XIX. Applying clinical trial results: A. How to use an article measuring the effect of an intervention on surrogate end points. JAMA 1999; 282:771–778.
13. Burtin P, Taddio A, Ariburnu O, et al. Safety of metronidazole in pregnancy: A meta-analysis. Am J Obstet Gynecol 1995; 172:525–529.
14. Carey JC, Klebanoff MA, Hauth JC, et al. Metronidazole to prevent preterm delivery in pregnant women with symptomatic bacterial vaginosis. N Engl J Med 2000; 342:534–540.
15. Carey MP, Kalra DL, Carey KB, et al. Stress and unaided smoking cessation: A prospective investigation. J Consult Clin Psychol 1993; 61:831–838.
16. Centers for Disease Control and Prevention. 1998 Guidelines for treatment of sexually transmitted diseases. MMWR Morb Mortal Wkly Rep 1998; 47:1–111.

17. Chan AW, Ross J. Management of unstable coronary syndromes in patients with previous coronary artery bypass grafts following coronary angiography. Clin Invest Med 1997; 20:320–326.
18. Cohen HA, Woloch B, Linder N, et al. J Fam Pract 1997; 44:290–292.
19. Colour vision screening: A critical appraisal of the literature. New Zealand Health Technology Assessment. p. 23, 26.
20. Dans AL, Dans LF, Guyatt GH, Richardson S. Users'guides to the medical literature: XIV. How to decide on the applicability of clinical trial results to your patient. Evidence Based Medicine Working Group. JAMA 1998; 279:545–549.
21. Dawes M, Davies P, Gray A, et al. Evidence-Based Practice: A Primer for Health Care Professionals. Churchill Livingstone; 1999.
22. Dick PT, Feldman W. Routine diagnostic imaging for childhood urinary tract infections: A systematic review. J Pediatr 1996; 128:15–22.
23. Drummond MF, Richardson WS, O'Brien BJ, et al. Users' guides to the medical literature: XIII. How to use an article on economic analysis of clinical practice: A. Are the results of the study valid? Evidence-Based Medicine Working Group. JAMA 1997; 277:1552–1557.
24. Dupuy A, Benchikhi H, Roujeau JC, et al. Risk factors for erysipelas of the leg (cellulitis): Case-control study. BMJ 1999; 318:1591–1594.
25. Feldman RD, Campbell N, Larochelle P, et al. 1999 Canadian recommendations for the management of hypertension. Can Med Assoc J 1999; 161(12 Suppl):S1–S17. Also available at http://www.cma.ca/cmaj/vol-161/issue-12/hypertension/hyper-e.htm.
26. Flather MD, Yusuf S, Kober L, et al. Long-term ACE-inhibitor therapy in patients with heart failure or left-ventricular dysfunction: A systematic review of data from individual patients. Lancet 2000; 355:1575–1581.
27. Flynn CA, Helwig AL, Meurer LN. Bacterial vaginosis in pregnancy and the risk of prematurity: A meta-analysis. J Fam Pract 1999; 48:885–892.
28. Fodor JG, Frohlich JJ, Genest JJG, McPherson PR, for the Working Group on Hypercholesterolemia and Other Dyslipidemias. Recommendations for the management and treatment of dyslipidemia. Can Med Assoc J 2000; 162:1441–1447.
29. Gaster B, Hirsch IB. The effects of improved glycemic control on complications in type 2 diabetes. Arch Intern Med 1998; 158:134–140.
30. Giacomini MK, Cook DJ. Users' guides to the medical literature: XXIII. Qualitative research in health care: A. Are the results of the study valid? JAMA 2000; 284:357–362.
31. Goetsch VL, Abel JL, Pope MK. The effects of stress, mood, and coping on blood glucose in NIDDM: A prospective pilot evaluation. Behav Res Ther 1994; 32:503–510.
32. Gorelick MH, Shaw KN. Screening tests for urinary tract infection in children: A meta-analysis. Pediatrics 1999; 104:1–7.
33. Guyatt GH, Naylor CD, Juniper E, et al. Users' guides to the medical literature: XII. How to use articles about health-related quality of life. Evidence-Based Medicine Working Group. JAMA 1997; 277:1232–1237.

34. Guyatt GH, Sackett DL, Cook DJ. Users' guides to the medical literature: II. How to use an article about therapy or prevention: A. Are the results of the study valid? JAMA 1993; 270:2598–2601.
35. Guyatt GH, Sackett DL, Cook DJ. Users' guides to the medical literature: II. How to use an article about therapy or prevention: B. What were the results and will they help me in caring for my patients? JAMA 1994; 271:59–63.
36. Guyatt GH, Sackett DL, Sinclair JC, et al. Users' guides to the medical literature: IX. A method for grading health care recommendations. JAMA 1995; 274:1800–1804.
37. Guyatt GH, Sinclair J, Cook DJ, Glasziou P. Users' guides to the medical literature: XVI. How to use a treatment recommendation. JAMA 1999; 281:1836–1843.
38. Hansson L, Zanchetti A, Caruthers G, et al. Effects of intensive blood-pressure lowering and low-dose aspirin in patients with hypertension: Principal results of the Hypertension Optimal Treatment (HOT) randomized trial. Lancet 1998; 351:1755–1762.
39. Hay EM, Oaterson SM, Lewis M, et al. Pragmatic randomized controlled trial of local corticosteroid injection and naproxen for treatment of lateral epicondylitis of elbow in primary care. BMJ 1999; 319:964–968.
40. Hayward RSA, Wilson MC, Tunis SR, et al. Users' guides to the medical literature: VIII. How to use clinical practice guidelines: A. Are the recommendations valid? JAMA 1995; 274:570–574.
41. Hemmelgarn B, Suissa S, Huang A, et al. Benzodiazepine use and the risk of motor vehicle crash in the elderly. JAMA 1997; 278:27–31.
42. Herlitz J, Brandrup-Wognsen G, Karlson BW, et al. Mortality, risk indicators of death, mode of death and symptoms of angina pectoris during 5 years after coronary artery bypass grafting in men and women. J Intern Med 2000; 247:500–506.
43. Hershow RC, Kalish LA, Sha B, et al. Hepatitis C virus infection in Chicago women with or at risk for HIV infection. Sexual Transm Dis 1998; 527–532.
44. Holbrook AM, Crowther R, Lotter A, et al. Meta-analysis of benzodiazepine use in the treatment of insomnia. Can Med Assoc J 2000; 162:225–233.
45. Hook EW, Hooton TM, Horton CA, et al. Microbiologic evaluation of cutaneous cellulitis in adults. Arch Intern Med 1986; 146:295–297.
46. Horowitz MJ, Siegel B, Holen A, et al. Diagnostic criteria for complicated grief disorder. Am J Psychiatry 1997; 154:905–910.
47. Hunt DL, Jaeschke R, McKibbon KA: Users' guides to the medical literature: XXI. Using electronic health information resources in evidence-based practice. Evidence-Based Medicine Working Group. JAMA 2000; 283: 1875–1879.
48. Jackson R. Updated New Zealand cardiovascular disease risk-benefit prediction guide. BMJ 2000; 320:709–710.
49. Jaeschke R, Gordon H, Guyatt G, Sackett DL. Users' guides to the medical literature: III. How to use an article about a diagnostic test: B. What are the results and will they help me in caring for my patients? JAMA 1994; 271:703–707.

50. Jaeschke R, Guyatt G, Sackett DL. Users' guides to the medical literature: III. How to use an article about a diagnostic test: A. Are the results of the study valid? JAMA 1994; 271:389–391.

51. Jick H, Kaye JA, Vasilakis-Scaramozza C, Jick SS. Risk of venous thromboembolism among users of third generation oral contraceptives compared with users of oral contraceptives with levonorgestrel before and after 1995: Cohort and case-control analysis. BMJ 2000; 321:1190–1195.

52. Kalon KL, Anderson KM, Kannel WB, et al. Survival after onset of congestive heart failure in Framingham Heart Study subjects. Circulation 1993; 88:107–115.

53. Kaul TK, Fields BL, Riggins LS, et al. Reinterventions for recurrent ischemic heart disease following a successful first re-do myocardial revascularization: predictors, indications and results. Cardiovasc Surg 1999; 7:363–369.

54. Khadra MH, Pickard RS, Charlton M, et al. A prospective analysis of 1,930 patients with hematuria to evaluate current diagnostic practice. J Urol 2000; 163:524–527.

55. Knatterud GL, Klimt CR, Levin ME, et al. Effects of hypoglycemic agents on vascular complications in patients with adult-onset diabetes. JAMA 1978; 240:37–42.

56. Knutsson S, Engberg IB. An evaluation of patients' quality of life before, 6 weeks, and 6 months after total hip replacement surgery. J Adv Nurs 1999; 30:1349–1359.

57. Kreder HJ, Williams JIW, Jaglal S, et al. Are complication rates for elective primary total hip arthroplasty in Ontario related to surgeon and Hospital volumes? Can J Surg 1998; 41:431–437.

58. Laupacis A, Wells G, Richardson S, Tugwell P. Users' guides to the medical literature: V. How to use an article about prognosis. JAMA 1994; 272:234–237.

59. Leese GP, Jung RT, Guthrie C, et al. Morbidity in patients on L-thyroxine: A comparison of those with a normal TSH to those with suppressed TSH. Clin Endocrinol 1992; 37:500–503.

60. Leipzig RM, Cumming RG, Tinetti ME. Drugs and falls in the elderly: A systematic review and meta-analysis: I. Psychotropic drugs. J Am Geriatr Soc 1999; 47:30–39.

61. Levine M, Walter S, Lee H, et al. Users' guides to the medical literature: IV. How to use an article about harm. JAMA 1994; 271:1615–1619.

62. Lewis J. Clean-catch versus urine collection pads: A prospective trial. Pediatr Nurs 1998; 10:15–16.

63. Liaw LCT, Nayar DM, Pedler SJ, Coulthard MG. Home collection of urine for culture from infants by three methods: Survey of parents' preferences and bacterial contamination rates. BMJ 2000; 320:1312–1313.

64. Lloyd CE, Dyer PH, Lancashire RJ, et al. Association between stress and glycemic control in adults with type 1 (insulin dependent) diabetes. Diabetes Care 1999; 22:1278–1283.

65. Macksood MJ, James RE. The scrotal mass: Cause and diagnosis. Am J Surg 1983; 145:297–299.

66. McAlister FA, Laupacis A, Wells GA, Sackett DL. Users' guides to the medical literature: XIX. Applying clinical trial results: B. Guidelines for deter-

mining whether a drug is exerting (more than) a class effect. JAMA 1999; 282:1371–1377.

67. McAlister FA, Straus SE, Guyatt GH, Haynes RB. Users' guides to the medical literature: XX. Integrating research evidence with the care of the individual patient. JAMA 2000; 283:2829–2836.

68. McGinn TG, Guyatt GH, Wyer PC, et al. Users' guides to the medical literature: XXII. How to use articles about clinical decision rules. JAMA 2000; 284:79–84.

69. Morin CM, Colecchi C, Stone J, et al. Behavioral and pharmacological therapies for late-life insomnia. JAMA 1999; 281:991–999.

70. Morin CM, Culbert JP, Schwartz SM. Nonpharmacological interventions for insomnia: A meta-analysis of treatment efficacy. Am J Psychiatry 1994; 151:1172–1180.

71. Mostofi FK. Testicular tumors: Epidemiologic, etiologic, and pathologic features. Cancer 1973; 32:1186–1201.

72. Mozurkewich EL, Hutton E. Elective repeat cesarean delivery versus trial of labor: A meta-analysis of the literature from 1989 to 1999. Am J Obstet Gynecol 2000; 183:1187–1197.

73. Murakami S, Igarashi T, Hara S, Shumazaki J. Strategies for asymptomatic microscopic hematuria: A prospective study of 1034 patients. J Urol 1990; 144:99–101.

74. Naylor CD, Guyatt GH. Users' guides to the medical literature: XI. How to use an article about a clinical utilization review. Evidence-Based Medicine Working Group. JAMA 1996; 275:1435–1439.

75. Naylor CD, Guyatt GH: Users' guides to the medical literature: X. How to use an article reporting variations in the outcomes of health services. Evidence-Based Medicine Working Group. JAMA 1996; 275:554–558.

76. O'Brien BJ, Heyland D, Richardson WS, et al. Users' guides to the medical literature: XIII. How to use an article on economic analysis of clinical practice: B. What are the results and will they help me in caring for my patients? Evidence-Based Medicine Working Group [published erratum appears in JAMA 1997 Oct 1; 278:1064]. JAMA 1997; 277:1802–1806.

77. Owen RT, Tyrer P. Benzodiazepine dependence: A review of the evidence. Drugs 1983; 25:385–398.

78. Oxman A, Sackett DL, Guyatt GH. Users' guides to the medical literature: I. How to get started. JAMA 1993; 270:2093–2095.

79. Oxman AD, Cook DJ, Guyatt GH. Users' guides to the medical literature: VI. How to use an overview. Evidence-Based Medicine Working Group. JAMA 1994; 272:1367–1371.

80. Parrott AC, Kaye FJ. Daily uplifts, hassles, stresses and cognitive failures: In cigarette smokers, abstaining smokers, and non-smokers. Behav Pharmacol 1999; 10:639–646.

81. Peters A, Ehlers M, Blank B, et al. Excess triiodothyronine as a risk factor for coronary events. 2000; 160:1993–1998.

82. Polak V, Hornak M. The value of scrotal ultrasound in patients with suspected testicular tumour. Int Urol Nephrol 1990; 20:467–473.

83. Randolph AG, Haynes RB, Wyatt JC, et al. Users guide to medical literature: XVIII. How to use an article evaluating the clinical impact of a

computer-based clinical decision support system. JAMA 1999; 282: 67–74.

84. Richardson WS, Detsky AS: Users' guides to the medical literature: VII. How to use a clinical decision analysis: A. Are the results of the study valid? JAMA 1995; 273:1292–1295.

85. Richardson WS, Detsky AS: Users' guides to the medical literature: VII. How to use a clinical decision analysis: B. What are the results and will they help me in caring for my patients? JAMA 1995; 273:1610–1613.

86. Richardson WS, Wilson MC, Guyatt GH, et al. Users' guides to the medical literature: XV. How to use an article about disease probability for differential diagnosis. JAMA 1999; 281:1214–1219.

87. Rodigro EK, King MB, Williams P. Health of long term benzodiazepine users. BMJ 1988; 296:603–606.

88. Romero R, Oyarzun E, Mazor M, et al. Meta-analysis of the relationship between asymptomatic bacteriuria and pre-term delivery/low birth weight. Obstet Gynecol 1989; 73:576–582.

89. Rozanski A, Blumenthal JA, Kaplan J. Impact of psychological factors on the pathogenesis of cardiovascular disease and implications for therapy. Circulation 1999; 99:2192–2217.

90. Sackett DL, Haynes RB, Guyatt GH, Tugwell P. Clinical Epidemiology: A Basic Science for Clinical Medicine. 2nd edition. Boston: Little, Brown; 1991.

91. Sackett DL, Strauss SE, Richardson WS, et al. Evidence Based Medicine: How to Practice and Reach EBM. 2nd edition. Churchill Livingstone; 2000.

92. Scandinavian Simvastatin Survival Study Group. Randomized trial of cholesterol lowering in 4444 patients with coronary heart disease: The Scandinavian Simvastatin Survival Study (4S). Lancet 1944; 344:1383–1389.

93. Shanfield SB, Benjamin H, Swain BJ. Parents reactions to the death of an adult child from cancer. Am J Psychiatry 1984; 141:1092–1094.

94. Sheldon F. ABC of palliative care: Bereavement. BMJ 1998; 216:456–458.

95. Shepherd J, Cobbe SM, Ford I, et al. Prevention of coronary heart disease with pravastatin in men with hypercholesterolemia. N Engl J Med 1995; 333:1301–1307.

96. Simpson RJ, Power KG, Wallace LA, et al. Controlled comparison of the characteristics of long-term benzodiazepine users in general practice. Br J Gen Pract 1990; 40:22–26.

97. Skinner JS, Farrer M, Albers CJ, et al. Patient-related outcomes five years after coronary artery bypass graft surgery. QJM 1999; 92:87–96.

98. Smaill F. Antibiotics for symptomatic bacteriuria in pregnancy. Cochrane review. In: The Cochrane Library, Issue 4. Oxford: Update Software; 2000.

99. Sparling PF. Gonococcal infections. In: Cecil's Textbook of Internal Medicine. MDConsult available at http://www.mdconsult.com.

100. Spence D, Barnett PA, Linden W, et al. Recommendations on stress management. 0Can Med Assoc J 1999; 160(9 Suppl):S46–S50.

101. Spencer J, Lindsell D, Mastorakou I. Ultrasonography compared with intravenous urography in the investigation of adults with haematuria. BMJ 1990; 301:1074–1076.

102. The Heart Outcomes Prevention Evaluation Study Investigators. Effects of an angiotension converting enzyme inhibitor, ramipril, on cardiovascular events in high-risk patients. N Engl J Med 2000; 342:145–153.
103. Torian LV, Makki HA, Menzies IB, et al. High HIV seroprevalence associated with gonorrhea: New York City Department of Health, sexually transmitted disease clinics, 1990–1997. AIDS 2000; 14:189–195.
104. Townsend. Sabiston Textbook of Surgery. 16th edition. Philadelphia: WB Saunders; p. 1690.
105. UK Prospective Diabetes Study Group. Intensive blood-glucose control with sulphonylureas or insulin compared with conventional treatment and risk of complications in patients with type 2 diabetes. Lancet 1998; 352:837–853.
106. UK Prospective Diabetes Study Group. Tight blood pressure control and risk of macrovascular and microvascular complications in type 2 diabetes: UKPDS 38. BMJ 1998; 317:703–713.
107. Veldhuyzen van Zanten SJO, Flook N, Chiba N, et al. An evidence-based approach to the management of uninvestigated dyspepsia in the era of *Helicobacter pylori.* Can Med Assoc J 2000; 162(12 Suppl):S3–S24.
108. Vrijkotte TGM, van Doornen LZP, de Geus EJC. Effects of work stress on ambulatory blood pressure, heart rate, and heart rate variability. Hypertension 2000; 35:880–886.
109. Walsh. Campbell's Urology. 7th edition. Philadelphia: WB Saunders; p. 143.
110. Wilson MC, Hayward RSA, Tunis SR, et al. Users' guides to the medical literature: VIII. How to use clinical practice guidelines: B. What are the recommendations and will they help you in caring for your patients? JAMA 1995; 274:1630–1632.
111. Wood-Baker R, Walters EH, Gibson P. Corticosteroids for acute exacerbations of chronic obstructive pulmonary disease. Cochrane Review. In: The Cochrane Library, Issue 1. Oxford: Update Software; 2001.
112. Wright JM, Lee CH, Chambers GK. Systematic review of antihypertensive therapies: Does the evidence assist in choosing a first-line drug? Can Med Assoc J 1999; 161:25–32.

Obtaining **MAINPRO-C** Credits

A family physician reading this book has the option of participating in an exercise that can be submitted to the College of Family Physicians of Canada (CFPC) for MAINPRO-C credits. The MAINPRO-C process requires that evidence or information be critically assessed, in the context of the physician's practice, to determine whether it can be appropriately applied to that physician's practice. A practice decision is made based on the critically appraised evidence, and a few months later the physician reflects on the effect of that decision on his or her practice. The design of this book facilitates this process for physicians using it for the purpose of MAINPRO-C credits. The clinical scenarios and questions are relevant to a family physician's practice, but the MAINPRO-C process requires that the reader consider the degree to which the scenario and the question fit with his or her own practice.

When completing your MAINPRO-C exercise, it is important that you look for other information that would address the clinical question to ensure that you have the best evidence to answer the question in the context of your practice and your patient. You may complete and submit a maximum of five MAINPRO-C forms. Each of the five reflective exercises is worth 2 MAINPRO-C credits for a maximum of 10 MAINPRO-C credits. Each reflective exercise must be based on 1 of the 43 clinical questions in the clinical scenarios in this book. Each reflective exercise must concern a different type of clinical question. There are five types of clinical questions in the book: diagnosis, therapy, harm, prognosis, and cause. They are described in the Preface.

The following table lists each of the 43 questions in this book and the type or types of questions they represent. Some of the questions have features of more than one of the five types of questions. You may choose which type of question you want them to represent, but any single question can be used only once.

Question Number	Question Type(s)	Question Number	Question Type(s)
1	Therapy/harm	23	Therapy/Prognosis
2	Therapy	24	Therapy/Prognosis
3	Cause	25	Therapy
4	Prognosis/harm/therapy	26	Prognosis
5	Therapy	27	Harm
6	Harm	28	Therapy/Harm
7	Therapy/cause	29	Prognosis
8	Therapy/harm	30	Prognosis
9	Prognosis/harm	31	Prognosis
10	Prognosis	32	Diagnosis/Prognosis
11	Therapy	33	Diagnosis
12	Cause	34	Diagnosis
13	Therapy	35	Diagnosis
14	Harm	36	Prognosis/harm
15	Diagnosis	37	Prognosis
16	Cause/therapy	38	Diagnosis
17	Diagnosis	39	Prognosis/diagnosis
18	Diagnosis	40	Therapy/harm
19	Harm	41	Prognosis/harm
20	Prognosis/cause	42	Therapy
21	Therapy	43	Diagnosis
22	Prognosis		

To claim your MAINPRO-C credit, complete the forms for the types of questions on which you wish to work. Tear them out and mail them directly to the College. Photocopies, scanned images, and faxed copies are not acceptable. You can verify that your credits have been accepted by checking your MAINPRO-C credit record online at *http://www.cfpc.ca/MAINPRO/MAINPRO.ASP.*

THE BEDFORD MYSTERY: AN EVIDENCE-BASED CLINICAL MYSTERY
Submission form for MAINPRO-C credits

This form documents how you used your experience with reading The Bedford Mystery: An Evidence-Based Clinical Mystery to reflect critically on new information and how you introduced it into your practice. It also documents your experience with the book as a model for the processes used in evidence-based medicine, including critical appraisal of the literature and the application of evidence to practice. You may complete and submit to the CFPC all or any of these forms for the reading and reflective activities you undertook during the process of working through this book. You will receive 2 MAINPRO-C credits for each satisfactorily completed form you submit. Each of the five forms concerns a different type of clinical question used in the book. There are five types of questions. These relate to diagnosis, therapy, harm, prognosis, and cause. This form should relate to a question of **DIAGNOSIS.**

Name: _____

Address: _____

City: _____ Province, state, or country:_____

Upon which question number in the book is this reflective learning exercise based? ___

Step 1: Formulate your practice question

First rewrite the question as asked in the book.

_____
_____
_____

Then, reformulate the question as it relates as directly as possible to your personal practice context and/or learning objectives.

_____
_____
_____

Step 2. Describe the information you reviewed

Describe the type and design of the study(s) reviewed by the authors of the book to answer this question. Consider whether the study(s) reflected research results or expert opinion. How well did the authors explore the available literature to answer this question with the best evidence?

_____
_____
_____
_____
_____
_____

What other sources of information or evidence did you use to understand better the question and/or learning objective?

Peer-reviewed articles	Peer-reviewed textbooks	Patient feedback
Non–peer-reviewed articles	Internet	Peers
Experts	Other_____	

Step 3: Consider the information

What is your assessment of the quality of the information that was reviewed in the book to answer this question? Was the assessment valid and relevant? How is it applicable to your practice? Do you agree with the assessment? If not, why not and how would you assess the information? What other information did you find that is more useful in addressing the question as it relates to your practice context?

_____

_____

_____

_____

_____

_____

_____

_____

_____

_____

_____

Step 4: Make a decision about your practice

Based on what you have learned, what decisions have you made about your practice and/or work?

_____

_____

_____

_____

_____

What must you do to integrate these decisions into your practice and/or work? What kinds of barriers/difficulties do you foresee?

_____

_____

_____

_____

_____

_____

_____

_____

Complete the following at least 2 months later.

Step 5: Evaluate/reflect on the impact of your decisions

Please describe your reflections on the impact this process has had on your practice and/or work. Consider questions such as:
- What impact has this process had on your practice generally?
- How do you feel now about the decision(s) you made?
- How successful have you been in incorporating them into your practice? What kinds of barriers have you confronted?
- What are you doing now that you didn't do before? What has happened to your confidence in this area?
- What kind of feedback have you received from your patients, staff, or colleagues?
- What new information have you seen? How has this further modified your approach? What further changes do you intend to make?
- What further areas of practice change, reassessment, and/or intervention have you identified? What plans do you have to address these?

_____
_____
_____
_____
_____
_____
_____
_____
_____
_____

Signature: _____   Date: _____

To claim your credits, send the completed original form to the CFPC by mail:
2630 Skymark Avenue, Mississauga, ON L4W 5A4

THE BEDFORD MYSTERY: AN EVIDENCE-BASED CLINICAL MYSTERY
Submission form for MAINPRO-C credits

> This form documents how you used your experience with reading The Bedford
> Mystery: An Evidence-Based Clinical Mystery to reflect critically on new
> information and how you introduced it into your practice. It also documents your
> experience with the book as a model for the processes used in evidence-based
> medicine, including critical appraisal of the literature and the application of
> evidence to practice. You may complete and submit to the CFPC all or any of
> these forms for the reading and reflective activities you undertook during the
> process of working through this book. You will receive 2 MAINPRO-C credits for
> each satisfactorily completed form you submit. Each of the five forms concerns a
> different type of clinical question used in the book. There are five types of
> questions. These relate to diagnosis, therapy, harm, prognosis, and cause. This
> form should relate to a question of **THERAPY.**

Name: _____

Address: _____

City: _____ Province, state, or country:_____

Upon which question number in the book is this reflective learning exercise based? ___

Step 1: Formulate your practice question

First rewrite the question as asked in the book.

_____

_____

_____

Then, reformulate the question as it relates as directly as possible to your personal practice context and/or learning objectives.

_____

_____

_____

Step 2. Describe the information you reviewed

Describe the type and design of the study(s) reviewed by the authors of the book to answer this question. Consider whether the study(s) reflected research results or expert opinion. How well did the authors explore the available literature to answer this question with
the best evidence?

_____

_____

_____

_____

_____

_____

What other sources of information or evidence did you use to understand better the question and/or learning objective?

Peer-reviewed articles	Peer-reviewed textbooks	Patient feedback
Non–peer-reviewed articles	Internet	Peers
Experts	Other_____	

Step 3: Consider the information

What is your assessment of the quality of the information that was reviewed in the book to answer this question? Was the assessment valid and relevant? How is it applicable to your practice? Do you agree with the assessment? If not, why not and how would you assess the information? What other information did you find that is more useful in addressing the question as it relates to your practice context?

_____

_____

_____

_____

_____

_____

_____

_____

_____

_____

Step 4: Make a decision about your practice

Based on what you have learned, what decisions have you made about your practice and/or work?

_____

_____

_____

_____

_____

What must you do to integrate these decisions into your practice and/or work? What kinds of barriers/difficulties do you foresee?

_____

_____

_____

_____

_____

_____

_____

Complete the following at least 2 months later.

Step 5: Evaluate/reflect on the impact of your decisions

Please describe your reflections on the impact this process has had on your practice and/or work. Consider questions such as:
- What impact has this process had on your practice generally?
- How do you feel now about the decision(s) you made?
- How successful have you been in incorporating them into your practice? What kinds of barriers have you confronted?
- What are you doing now that you didn't do before? What has happened to your confidence in this area?
- What kind of feedback have you received from your patients, staff, or colleagues?
- What new information have you seen? How has this further modified your approach? What further changes do you intend to make?
- What further areas of practice change, reassessment, and/or intervention have you identified? What plans do you have to address these?

_____

_____

_____

_____

_____

_____

_____

_____

_____

_____

Signature: _____   Date: _____

To claim your credits, send the completed original form to the CFPC by mail:
2630 Skymark Avenue, Mississauga, ON L4W 5A4

THE BEDFORD MYSTERY: AN EVIDENCE-BASED CLINICAL MYSTERY
Submission form for MAINPRO-C credits

This form documents how you used your experience with reading <u>The Bedford Mystery: An Evidence-Based Clinical Mystery</u> to reflect critically on new information and how you introduced it into your practice. It also documents your experience with the book as a model for the processes used in evidence-based medicine, including critical appraisal of the literature and the application of evidence to practice. You may complete and submit to the CFPC all or any of these forms for the reading and reflective activities you undertook during the process of working through this book. You will receive 2 MAINPRO-C credits for each satisfactorily completed form you submit. Each of the five forms concerns a different type of clinical question used in the book. There are five types of questions. These relate to diagnosis, therapy, harm, prognosis, and cause. This form should relate to a question of **HARM.**

Name: _____

Address: _____

City: _____ Province, state, or country:_____

Upon which question number in the book is this reflective learning exercise based? ___

Step 1: Formulate your practice question

First rewrite the question as asked in the book.

_____

_____

_____

Then, reformulate the question as it relates as directly as possible to your personal practice context and/or learning objectives.

_____

_____

_____

Step 2. Describe the information you reviewed

Describe the type and design of the study(s) reviewed by the authors of the book to answer this question. Consider whether the study(s) reflected research results or expert opinion. How well did the authors explore the available literature to answer this question with the best evidence?

_____

_____

_____

_____

_____

What other sources of information or evidence did you use to understand better the question and/or learning objective?

Peer-reviewed articles	Peer-reviewed textbooks	Patient feedback
Non–peer-reviewed articles	Internet	Peers
Experts	Other_____	

Step 3: Consider the information

What is your assessment of the quality of the information that was reviewed in the book to answer this question? Was the assessment valid and relevant? How is it applicable to your practice? Do you agree with the assessment? If not, why not and how would you assess the information? What other information did you find that is more useful in addressing the question as it relates to your practice context?

_____

_____

_____

_____

_____

_____

_____

_____

_____

_____

Step 4: Make a decision about your practice

Based on what you have learned, what decisions have you made about your practice and/or work?

_____

_____

_____

_____

_____

What must you do to integrate these decisions into your practice and/or work? What kinds of barriers/difficulties do you foresee?

_____

_____

_____

_____

_____

_____

_____

Complete the following at least 2 months later.

Step 5: Evaluate/reflect on the impact of your decisions

Please describe your reflections on the impact this process has had on your practice and/or work. Consider questions such as:

- What impact has this process had on your practice generally?
- How do you feel now about the decision(s) you made?
- How successful have you been in incorporating them into your practice? What kinds of barriers have you confronted?
- What are you doing now that you didn't do before? What has happened to your confidence in this area?
- What kind of feedback have you received from your patients, staff, or colleagues?
- What new information have you seen? How has this further modified your approach? What further changes do you intend to make?
- What further areas of practice change, reassessment, and/or intervention have you identified? What plans do you have to address these?

_____

_____

_____

_____

_____

_____

_____

_____

_____

_____

Signature: _____ Date: _____

To claim your credits, send the completed original form to the CFPC by mail:
2630 Skymark Avenue, Mississauga, ON L4W 5A4

THE BEDFORD MYSTERY: AN EVIDENCE-BASED CLINICAL MYSTERY
Submission form for MAINPRO-C credits

> This form documents how you used your experience with reading The Bedford Mystery: An Evidence-Based Clinical Mystery to reflect critically on new information and how you introduced it into your practice. It also documents your experience with the book as a model for the processes used in evidence-based medicine, including critical appraisal of the literature and the application of evidence to practice. You may complete and submit to the CFPC all or any of these forms for the reading and reflective activities you undertook during the process of working through this book. You will receive 2 MAINPRO-C credits for each satisfactorily completed form you submit. Each of the five forms concerns a different type of clinical question used in the book. There are five types of questions. These relate to diagnosis, therapy, harm, prognosis, and cause. This form should relate to a question of **PROGNOSIS.**

Name: _____

Address: _____

City: _____ Province, state, or country:_____

Upon which question number in the book is this reflective learning exercise based? ___

Step 1: Formulate your practice question

First rewrite the question as asked in the book.

_____
_____
_____

Then, reformulate the question as it relates as directly as possible to your personal practice context and/or learning objectives.

_____
_____
_____

Step 2. Describe the information you reviewed

Describe the type and design of the study(s) reviewed by the authors of the book to answer this question. Consider whether the study(s) reflected research results or expert opinion. How well did the authors explore the available literature to answer this question with the best evidence?

_____
_____
_____
_____
_____
_____
_____

What other sources of information or evidence did you use to understand better the question and/or learning objective?

Peer-reviewed articles	Peer-reviewed textbooks	Patient feedback
Non–peer-reviewed articles	Internet	Peers
Experts	Other_____	

Step 3: Consider the information

What is your assessment of the quality of the information that was reviewed in the book to answer this question? Was the assessment valid and relevant? How is it applicable to your practice? Do you agree with the assessment? If not, why not and how would you assess the information? What other information did you find that is more useful in addressing the question as it relates to your practice context?

_____
_____
_____
_____
_____
_____
_____
_____
_____
_____
_____

Step 4: Make a decision about your practice

Based on what you have learned, what decisions have you made about your practice and/or work?

_____
_____
_____
_____
_____

What must you do to integrate these decisions into your practice and/or work? What kinds of barriers/difficulties do you foresee?

_____
_____
_____
_____
_____
_____

Complete the following at least 2 months later.

Step 5: Evaluate/reflect on the impact of your decisions

Please describe your reflections on the impact this process has had on your practice and/or work. Consider questions such as:

- What impact has this process had on your practice generally?
- How do you feel now about the decision(s) you made?
- How successful have you been in incorporating them into your practice? What kinds of barriers have you confronted?
- What are you doing now that you didn't do before? What has happened to your confidence in this area?
- What kind of feedback have you received from your patients, staff, or colleagues?
- What new information have you seen? How has this further modified your approach? What further changes do you intend to make?
- What further areas of practice change, reassessment, and/or intervention have you identified? What plans do you have to address these?

_____

_____

_____

_____

_____

_____

_____

_____

_____

_____

Signature: _____   Date: _____

To claim your credits, send the completed original form to the CFPC by mail:
2630 Skymark Avenue, Mississauga, ON L4W 5A4

THE BEDFORD MYSTERY: AN EVIDENCE-BASED CLINICAL MYSTERY
Submission form for MAINPRO-C credits

This form documents how you used your experience with reading <u>The Bedford Mystery: An Evidence-Based Clinical Mystery</u> to reflect critically on new information and how you introduced it into your practice. It also documents your experience with the book as a model for the processes used in evidence-based medicine, including critical appraisal of the literature and the application of evidence to practice. You may complete and submit to the CFPC all or any of these forms for the reading and reflective activities you undertook during the process of working through this book. You will receive 2 MAINPRO-C credits for each satisfactorily completed form you submit. Each of the five forms concerns a different type of clinical question used in the book. There are five types of questions. These relate to diagnosis, therapy, harm, prognosis, and cause. This form should relate to a question of **CAUSE.**

Name: _____

Address: _____

City: _____ Province, state, or country:_____

Upon which question number in the book is this reflective learning exercise based? ___

Step 1: Formulate your practice question

First rewrite the question as asked in the book.

_____
_____
_____

Then, reformulate the question as it relates as directly as possible to your personal practice context and/or learning objectives.

_____
_____
_____

Step 2. Describe the information you reviewed

Describe the type and design of the study(s) reviewed by the authors of the book to answer this question. Consider whether the study(s) reflected research results or expert opinion. How well did the authors explore the available literature to answer this question with the best evidence?

_____
_____
_____
_____
_____
_____
_____

What other sources of information or evidence did you use to understand better the question and/or learning objective?

Peer-reviewed articles	Peer-reviewed textbooks	Patient feedback
Non–peer-reviewed articles	Internet	Peers
Experts	Other_____	

Step 3: Consider the information

What is your assessment of the quality of the information that was reviewed in the book to answer this question? Was the assessment valid and relevant? How is it applicable to your practice? Do you agree with the assessment? If not, why not and how would you assess the information? What other information did you find that is more useful in addressing the question as it relates to your practice context?

_____

_____

_____

_____

_____

_____

_____

_____

_____

_____

_____

Step 4: Make a decision about your practice

Based on what you have learned, what decisions have you made about your practice and/or work?

_____

_____

_____

_____

_____

What must you do to integrate these decisions into your practice and/or work? What kinds of barriers/difficulties do you foresee?

_____

_____

_____

_____

_____

_____

_____

Complete the following at least 2 months later.

Step 5: Evaluate/reflect on the impact of your decisions

Please describe your reflections on the impact this process has had on your practice and/or work. Consider questions such as:

- What impact has this process had on your practice generally?
- How do you feel now about the decision(s) you made?
- How successful have you been in incorporating them into your practice? What kinds of barriers have you confronted?
- What are you doing now that you didn't do before? What has happened to your confidence in this area?
- What kind of feedback have you received from your patients, staff, or colleagues?
- What new information have you seen? How has this further modified your approach? What further changes do you intend to make?
- What further areas of practice change, reassessment, and/or intervention have you identified? What plans do you have to address these?

_____

_____

_____

_____

_____

_____

_____

_____

_____

_____

Signature: _____   Date: _____

To claim your credits, send the completed original form to the CFPC by mail:
2630 Skymark Avenue, Mississauga, ON L4W 5A4

INDEX

Caruncles, urethral, hematuria associated
  with, 48
Case-control, 151
Case-series, 151
Cellulitis, 43–44, 45–46
CER (control event rate), 148, 149, 152
Cerivastatin (Baycol), removal from mar-
  ket, 31
Cervicitis, gonococcal, 104–105
Cesarean section
  trial of labor prior to, 11, 13–15
    meta-analysis of, 148–150
  vaginal birth after, 12, 13–15
Characters
  Collier, Mary, 139–142
  FitzPatrick, Sean, 56, 58, 71–78, 99,
    100, 101, 107–111, 114, 131,
    146
  Hagarty, John, 93–97
  Harris, Jane, 135–137
  Hynes, Joey, 113, 114, 131–133
  Kelland, Janet, 53
  Kelland, Larry, 53
  Ling, Jenny, 99–100, 143, 145, 146
  Nash, Leo, 103, 113, 114, 131–133,
    145–146
  Nelson, Leonard, 143–144, 145–146
  Richard, Stefan, 65–66, 113
  Sampson, Alexander, 1, 2, 11, 25–38,
    39, 54, 83–86, 87, 100, 101, 103,
    134
  Sampson, Cecelia, 1–9, 11, 25, 39, 54,
    79–81, 103, 134
  Sampson, Joanne, 1, 26, 53, 54, 100,
    101, 134
  Sampson, Martin, 39, 43
  Sampson, Nicholas, 1, 2, 11, 12, 25,
    39, 53–56, 65, 66, 71, 72, 79,
    83–84, 87, 88, 99, 100, 131, 132,
    133, 134
  Sampson-Savoy, Nancy, 1, 39–42, 43,
    54, 83, 101, 103–106, 132, 134, ix
  Savoy, Maurice, 66, 101
  Savoy, Pierre, 1, 2, 11, 25, 39, 43–46,
    54, 66, 71, 79, 87, 88, 100, 101,
    103, 106, 107, 113, 131–133
  Simms, Gemma, 119–126
  Simms, Mr., 119, 126
  Simple, Jonathon, 56
  Slade, Derrick, 83, 87, 100
  Starkes, Cecil, 47–51

  Stenson, Robert, 65–66, 100, 113–117
  Stephens, Amy, 11, 12, 54, 55–56,
    57–58, 66, 71, 72, 79, 83, 99,
    100, 103, 131–132, 133
  Stephens, Beatrice, 56, 57–64
  Stephens, Tom, 57
  Walters, Joan, 65–70, 99
  Walters, Matt, 65
  Walters-Sampson, Harry, 11
  Walters-Sampson, Joanne, 11–24, 65,
    87–91
  Wells, Gerald, 53
  Werston, Simon, 127–129
Children, urinary tract infections in,
    119–126
  antibiotic prophylaxis against,
    124–125
  diagnostic sampling in, 123–125
  nitrate dipstick sampling in, 119–121
  renal scarring associated with, 125
  urinary tract abnormalities associated
    with, 123–125
  urine sampling in, 119, 120,
    121–122
Chlorpropamide, 3, 4
Cholesterol, as coronary events risk fac-
  tor, 85, 86
Chronic obstructive pulmonary disease
  (COPD)
  acute exacerbations of, 139–142
  steroid therapy for, 141–142
CI (confidence interval), 151–152
Cisapride
  as cardiac mortality cause, 127
  removal from market, 129
Cloxacillin, 46
Cochrane Collaboration, 17–19, 22–24,
    151
Co-codamol, as lateral epicondylitis treat-
  ment, 95
Cohort study, 151
Colorblindness
  detection of, 143–144
  as motor vehicle accident risk factor,
    119, 120, 126
Complicated grief disorder, 63, 64
Confidence interval (CI), 151–152
Confounding variable, 152
Congenital malformations
  metronidazole-related, 20–21
  vitamin A-related, 87–91

Nonsteroidal anti-inflammatory drugs
  as gastrointestinal hemorrhage cause,
    41
  as lateral epicondylitis treatment, 93,
    95–96
Number-needed-to-treat (NNT), 148, 150,
    153

O
Obesity, as cardiovascular disease risk
    factor, 25, 27
Odds, 153
Odds ratio (OR), 148, 153
Oral contraceptives, as deep vein throm-
    bosis risk factor, 39–42
Oral hypoglyemic agents, 1, 2, 3–4
OR (odds ratio), 148
Ottawa Ankle Rules, 43, 44–45, 150
Overview, 153

P
Pain, lateral epicondylitis-related, 93–97
Pap smear, 39
Parents, of deceased adult children, 62
Patient expected event rate (PEER), 153
Pelvic inflammatory disease, gonococcal
    cervicitis-related, 104–105
Peripheral vascular disease, diabetes
    mellitus-related, 80
Peto odds ratio, 148, 149
Physical examination, exposure and in-
    spection during, 43
Placebo, 153
Positive predictive value, 153
Posttest probability, 153
Potassium supplementation, in hyperten-
    sion, 25
Practice guidelines, clinical, 151
Pregnancy, 11–24
  bacterial vaginosis during, 12, 15–22
  vitamin A supplementation during,
    87–91
Premature delivery
  bacterial vaginosis-related, 15–16, 17,
    18–20, 21–22
  maternal bacteriuria-related, 23, 24
Premature rupture of membranes, bacter-
    ial vaginosis-related, 17, 18, 19,
    21–22
Pretest probability, 153
Prevalence, 153

Prokinetic agents, 127, 128, 129
Prostate cancer, asymptomatic hematuria
    associated with, 50
Proton-pump inhibitors, 129
Psychological factors, in coronary artery
    disease, 36
Publication bias, 153
Puncture wounds, 43–44
Pyelography, intravenous, for asympto-
    matic hematuria evaluation, 48,
    49, 51
Pyelonephritis
  in children, 123, 124
  during pregnancy, 23, 24

Q
Quality of life, of hip replacement pa-
    tients, 136–137
Quazepam, 5

R
Ramipril
  cardioprotective effects of, 27, 35–36
  as congestive heart failure treatment,
    67, 68, 70
  use in diabetics, 35–36, 79
Randomized controlled trials, 147–148,
    153
Ranitidine, as gastroesophageal reflux
    treatment, 127, 129
RCTs. See Randomized controlled trials
Reference standard, 153
Relative risk (RR), 148
Relative risk reduction (RRR), 154
Renal cancer, asymptomatic hematuria
    associated with, 50
Renal scarring, urinary tract infection-
    related, 125
Retinoic acid, 89
Retinol, 89
Retinopathy, diabetic, 4
Rhabdomyolysis, statins-related, 31
Risk, 154
Risk ratio (RR), 154
RR (relative risk), 148
RR (risk ratio), 154
RRR (relative risk reduction), 154

S
SAVE (Survival and Ventricular Enlarge-
    ment) trial, 67

Urinary tract infections
    asymptomatic hematuria associated
        with, 48, 50
    in children, 119–126
        antibiotic prophylaxis against,
            124–125
        diagnostic imaging in, 123–125
        nitrate dipstick testing in,
            119–121
        renal scarring associated with,
            125
        urinary tract abnormalities associated
            with, 123–125
        urine sampling in, 119, 120,
            121–122
Urine culture, for asymptomatic hema-
    turia evaluation, 47, 48, 49
Urine sampling, in children, 119, 120,
    121–122
Urologic cancer, hematuria associated
    with, 48
Urothelial cancer, asymptomatic hema-
    turia associated with, 50, 51
Uterus, cesarean section-related rupture
    of, 13, 14
    meta-analysis of, 148–150

V
Vaginal swabs, use in pregnant women,
    12, 22

Vaginosis, bacterial, during pregnancy,
    12, 15–22
    antibiotic treatment for, 15
    as low-birth-weight risk factor, 17, 18,
        19, 21–22
    as premature delivery risk factor,
        15–16, 17, 18–20, 21–22
    as premature rupture of membranes risk
        factor, 17, 18, 21–22
Valvular heart disease, congestive heart
    disease associated with, 69
Varicoceles, 114
Ventolin. See Albuterol
Vesicoureteral reflux
    in children, 123, 124–125
    hematuria associated with, 48
Vitamin A, teratogenicity of, 87–91
Vulvitis, 119

W
Weight loss, gastroesophageal reflux-
    related, 127
Women, cardiovascular disease risk as-
    sessment in, 34
Work stress, effect on ambulatory blood
    pressure, 36–37
Wounds, cellulitis of, 45

X
X-rays, of ankle injuries, 43, 44–45